Color Atlas of
COSMETIC OCULOFACIAL SURGERY

Commissioning Editor: **Paul Fam**
Project Development Manager: **Shuet-Kei Cheung**
Project Manager: **Glenys Norquay**
Illustration Manager: **Mick Ruddy**
Designer: **Andy Chapman**
Illustrator: **Linda Warren and Jenni Miller**
Page Layout: **Alan Palfreyman** (PTU Elsevier)

Color Atlas of
COSMETIC OCULOFACIAL SURGERY

William PD Chen MD FACS
Associate Clinical Professor of Ophthalmology
UCLA School of Medicine, Los Angeles, California; and
Ophthalmic Plastic Surgery Service
Harbor-UCLA Medical Center
Torrance, California
USA

Jemshed A Khan MD
Clinical Professor of Ophthalmology
Kansas University School of Medicine
Kansas City, Kansas
USA

Clinton D McCord Jr MD
Paces Plastic Surgery, Atlanta
Associate Clinical Professor of Plastic Surgery
Emory University School of Medicine
Atlanta, Georgia
USA

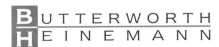

BUTTERWORTH
HEINEMANN

An imprint of Elsevier Inc

Philadelphia ● Edinburgh ● London ● New York ● Oxford ● St Louis ● Sydney ● Toronto ● 2004

BUTTERWORTH-HEINEMANN
An imprint of Elsevier Inc

First published 2004

ISBN 0 7506 7422 9

British Library Cataloguing in Publication Data
A catalogue record for this book is available from the British Library

Library of Congress Cataloging in Publication Data
A catalog record for this book is available from the Library of Congress

Notice
Medical knowledge is constantly changing. Standard safety precautions must be followed, but as new research and clinical experience broaden our knowledge, changes in treatment and drug therapy may become necessary or appropriate. Readers are advised to check the most current product information provided by the manufacturer of each drug to be administered to verify the recommended dose, the method and duration of administration, and contraindications. It is the responsibility of the practitioner, relying on experience and knowledge of the patient, to determine dosages and the best treatment for each individual patient. Neither the Publisher nor the authors assume any liability for any injury and/or damage to persons or property arising from this publication. The Publisher

Printed in China

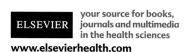

your source for books,
journals and multimedia
in the health sciences

www.elsevierhealth.com

The
Publisher's
policy is to use
**paper manufactured
from sustainable forests**

Contents

Preface

This project, *Color Atlas of Cosmetic Oculofacial Surgery*, is a joint effort of three authors, William Chen from Southern California, Jem Khan from Kansas City, Missouri and Clinton D McCord Jr of Atlanta, Georgia. All three are oculoplastic surgeons in private practices with cosmetic emphasis and each hold university clinical faculty appointments. Their combined efforts in covering this very specific field allows each author to delve into the fine details and nuances of various cosmetic surgeries as practiced now by oculoplastic as well as plastic surgeons with training from diverse backgrounds.

The format of the book adapts the forms of a practical color atlas as well as a teaching manual. The images are arranged such that the text on the page corresponds to them, and they are paired with specific comments including 'Pearls' and 'Pitfalls' when appropriate. Certain images have accompanying line drawings to clarify corresponding details. Tables and outlines as well as flow diagrams are used to present information and summaries in a succinct fashion. The book can be used as a learning text as well as a companion manual in an operating room setting. The readership pool would include practitioners in the field of plastic surgery, ophthalmology, head and neck surgery as well as facial plastic surgeons, and dermatologists who perform cosmetic surgery. The level of writing and the information conveyed are such that it will be of interest to sub-specialists like oculoplastic surgeons, and to specialists and house-officers in training.

The book covers the forehead and eyebrows (endoscopic surgery and direct browlift procedures), followed by upper eyelid blepharoplasty and lower eyelid blepharoplasty. Practitioners will find that there are specific needs one faces with each individual patient and therefore in the chapter on lower blepharoplasty, both the traditional skin-muscle flap, infraciliary approach and the more advanced cheek-lift (combined with lower blepharoplasty) are covered. The second half of the book covers laser blepharoplasty of the upper and lower eyelids, and laser resurfacing of the face and neck. Botox facial rejuvenation and ptosis repair are also covered. In addition, the highly specialized topic of Asian blepharoplasty, its method as practiced by Chen and re-operative challenges in upper lids of Asians have been completely updated in two comprehensive chapters, with pre-operative assessments in the form of hand drawings and images, as well as intraoperative findings and comments.

From the beginning, it has been a pleasure for me to participate in this project, being teamed with the capable and professional group at Elsevier. Our team members include Natasha Andjelkovic in Philadelphia; Paul Fam, Shuet-Kei Cheung, Firiel Benson and the developmental and copy-editing staff in London, as well as Glenys Norquay (Project Manager) in Edinburgh, Scotland. I am indebted to each of them for their tireless guidance along the development of this text, as well providing valuable feedback to me and to my co-authors. I would like to thank the graphic art crew at Elsevier for providing their expertise, and to Linda Warren, a medical artist in Austin, Texas for working with me on this project.

I wish to thank my friends and colleagues Jem Khan and Dr Sonny McCord for their generosity in participating in this project. I have learnt much from them.

William PD Chen
2004

Dedications

To my parents, Fred and Katie.
William PD Chen

To my wife, Michelle, and my sons, Alex, Corey, and Christopher.
Jemshed A Khan

To my family.
Clinton D McCord Jr

Examination and Interactions with Aesthetic Patients

Chapter 1

William PD Chen and Jemshed A Khan

Dr Chen's viewpoint

Cosmetic blepharoplasty is one of the most popular forms of aesthetic surgery of the face. The surgical outcome is intimately related to the interaction of the upper eyelids with the forehead and brows, as well as the lower eyelids, lateral canthi, and the midface and cheek's topography. Therefore, in any discussion and examination of a patient concerning this form of surgery, an astute clinician should consider the entire face, and not confine attention to only the superficial upper and lower eyelid skin layers. This awareness of surrounding as well as deeper structures will ultimately yield much better surgical outcome and a happier patient.

In my initial office consultation with a new patient, I first listen to his or her complaints, and mentally classify these into relative orders (or wish list) of which include those that can be improved upon, versus transient improvement or no improvement at all. I then assess from the patient's personality and temperament the degree of enthusiasm or tolerance to surgery he or she possesses. Ultimately, the surgeon and the patient need to mutually agree on what is comfortable, beneficial, and worthwhile for the patient to undertake. This may include financial matters, time commitment as to postoperative healing course, as well as overall general medical conditions that may have a bearing on the type of surgery and anesthesia recommended.

I always try to encourage patients to speak their mind, even if they may be embarrassed, and I try to facilitate this in an environment free of stress. Very often, patients may be overly self-conscious about an issue that matters very little to anyone they interact with, or the surgeon may need to point out an extreme condition that requires correction before the aesthetic outcome can be achieved, such as involutional ptosis in conjunction with upper eyelid hooding. It is important to customize individual aspects of your particular technique for that patient. For example, I have not performed two exactly identical procedures among any of my patients who have come to me to have Asian blepharoplasty.

After an adequate prioritization of goals with the patient, I then explain what the procedure involves, before, during, and after the surgery, and what is expected of the patient. This includes the mandatory preoperative cessation of aspirin products, non-steroidal anti-inflammatory drugs, as well as anticoagulants like coumadin and heparin.

The patients need to be quizzed as to whether they are taking any herbal formulas, ginseng compounds, or herbal teas, which frequently may contain therapeutics with anticoagulative properties ('circulatory-promoting, blood-flow-promoting' ingredients in traditional Chinese medicine).

The patient is given a detailed written list of preoperative and postoperative instructions with regard to bed rest during the first day, use of ice compresses as well as antibiotic ointments, what to expect, and instructions to call me should there be any unexpected outcome or medical emergency. The office staff are trained to make a follow-up telephone call to the patient the day after surgery, both to verify that the patient is stable and to confirm a return date for suture removal.

In the office chart for the patient, I record particular aspects of his or her facial structure (ptosis, ectropion, entropion, lateral canthal dehiscence, thinning of levator and aponeurosis, forehead brow over-action, prominent sulcus) (**Fig. 1.1**), what was mentioned to the patient (for example, one upper lid margin is half a millimeter lower than the other, one eye is more sunken and shows a more prominent sulcus), the patient's response and preferences (high crease, low crease, shape of crease line selected), as well as skin texture and pre-existent thinning of lower lid skin and telangiectatic blood vessels observed, plus what I tell patients as to whether their stated preferences could be achieved (**Fig. 1.2**). If a patient has thick dry skin, or oily complexion, superficial furuncles, or rosacea, these are all noted on my plan of management for this patient (**Fig. 1.3**).

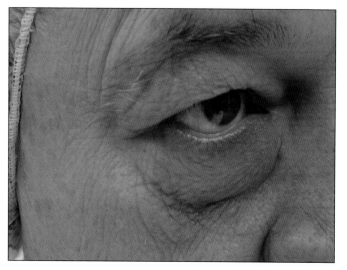

Figure 1.1 Elderly man with lower lid ectropion and cheek ptosis.

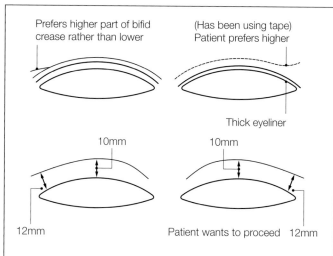

Figure 1.2 Actual drawing of patient's clinical findings on medical records.

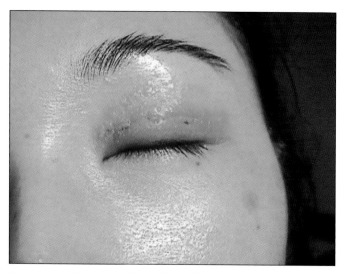

Figure 1.3 Asian female with eyelid cellulitis.

Postoperative dietary recommendations are also offered to facilitate uneventful and non-inflammatory healing of the skin (this is an aspect of traditional Chinese medicine that bewilders Western medical practitioners somewhat).

In California, informed consent for surgery is mandatory and we implement it in the office as well as in the outpatient surgical facilities. All aesthetic patients – for that matter, all patients in my offices – must have adequate photographic documentation of their current conditions. Typically, this includes a frontal view, oblique side views, upgaze and down-gaze, and, most importantly if the patient has had

previous surgeries, a close-up macro view of the existent surgical lines or lid-crease scar. This last item has been extremely useful for fully informing the patients in many of the revision cases that I have performed. In this very litigious climate, adequate documentation is truly the best policy.

As regards photographic media, I have shifted to digital photography since 1997. I use a Sony Mavica camera which take images in the 800×600 pixels range and stores them on flat 3.5-inch floppy disks (cost less than 30 cents each). The disk is conveniently kept in each patient's chart and can be used for preparing simple Powerpoint presentations for teaching purposes and community lectures (**Fig. 1.4**). I use two other higher-resolution cameras for more detailed images of selective conditions when I need them for publication purposes. The cameras are a Sony Cybershot with 3 megapixels and a Nikon Coolpix with 2 megapixels capabilities. I still keep my Kodachrome color slides collection accumulated over the last 20-plus years of practice.

If a patient appears extremely nervous, I usually try to call them the night before the procedure, to make sure all is well. On the day of surgery, in the preoperative area, I greet patients again and reiterate the goal(s) of the surgery. If there is any discrepancy between what I told the patient and what they think and expect of the surgery, I would always defer the surgery until another day, although this is extremely rare.

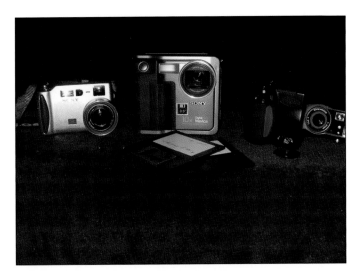

Figure 1.4 Digital cameras. In the center is a Sony Mavica that uses floppy disks for storage; to the left is a Sony Cybershot camera that uses memory sticks; to the right is a Nikon Coolpix 950 that uses compact flash memory cards.

Dr Khan's viewpoint

Several critical issues should be resolved during the preoperative consultation with a patient who desires aesthetic periocular surgery. The present discussion will focus narrowly on only those issues unique to aesthetic patients. First and foremost, the surgeon should elicit from the patient a designation of those specific topographic facial features that the patient would wish improved. Oftentimes, patients express concern that their periocular facial features are communicating unintended signals such as disapproval (glabellar frown lines), tiredness (lower eyelid fat pad herniation or upper eyelid ptosis), worry or aging (crow's-feet). Otherwise stated, the face is malfunctioning as an organ of communication.[1]

After ascertaining and documenting the patient's concerns as well as recording photographic appearance, the surgeon should evaluate the facial features for the anatomic basis of the patient's concerns. Many times, the patient's concerns are related to familial, gravitational, or age-related facial changes. The examination should also search for concurrent facial conditions that may complicate management of the patient's concerns. For example, herniating lower eyelid fat pads may be accompanied by festoons, periocular skin pigmentation, tear-trough deformity, midface descent, malar edema, skin wrinkling, and horizontal eyelid laxity. In the upper eyelids, complicating factors may include eyebrow ptosis, secondary eyebrow elevation, eyelid ptosis, lagophthalmos, prolapse of the lacrimal glands, asymmetrical eyelid creases or folds, and prominent retro-orbicularis oculi fat (ROOF). Documentation of the examination includes notation of any complicating facial features or findings.

The next step is for the surgeon to educate the patient regarding the anatomic basis for the patient's concerns as well as any relevant concurrent conditions. From this discussion one can proceed to outline the range of surgical options available that address the underlying anatomic causes of the patient's concerns. One should actively solicit and receive the patient's feedback as to which options best meet the patient's needs. During this portion of the discussion it is critical that the surgeon clearly establishes, in the patient's mind, reasonable postoperative expectations as to the degree of surgical improvement associated with the various surgical options. Patients who cannot accept a 'marked definite and noticeable improvement' as opposed to a 'perfect result' are sometimes poor candidates for aesthetic surgery. Informed consent regarding the risks, consequences, benefits, and alternatives of surgery consists of both a discussion with the patient as well as a signed consent document.

Finally, it is important to keep in mind that properly informed patients will not, and should not, always choose the surgical option that most effectively addresses their physical concerns. This is because the patient must also factor in other considerations, including cost, invasiveness, surgical risk, the location and visibility of surgical incisions, recovery times, postoperative morbidity, and procedure length. Indeed, the goal is not to invariably create the best aesthetic improvement, but rather to educate the patients to the point that they can select those procedures which best meet the patient's aesthetic goals while also respecting the patient's financial constraints, tolerance for surgical risk, and desires regarding rapidity of recovery.

REFERENCE

1. Khan JA. Aesthetic surgery: diagnosing and healing the miscues of human facial expression. Ophthal Plast Reconstr Surg 2001;17:4–6.

Eyelid Anatomy

William PD Chen, Jemshed A Khan, and Clinton D McCord Jr

Chapter 2

Upper Eyelid of Asians Without Crease

Approximately half of all Asians have some form of an upper eyelid crease; thus, there are about 50% of Asians who do not have a crease. This seems to affect most Asians of Han origin, including the Chinese, Koreans, Japanese, and China's minority tribes. The incidence within any given family appears to parallel the above statistic in that I often elicit the history that one of the parents has an upper lid crease whereas the other parent does not, and this also seems to hold true among the siblings.

In the past, the stereotypic conclusion that all Asians are without an upper eyelid crease may stem from the fact that Western plastic surgeons often may get to examine only those Asians who have no crease and therefore seek their services, although many do not.

We will describe some of the commonly observed features in Asians who do not have a crease, and also, among the Asians who do have a crease, what crease shape and size these tend to be (**Figs 2.1 & 2.2**).

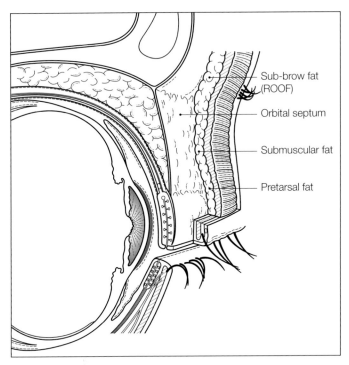

Figure 2.1 Cross-section of Asian upper eyelid without crease. (Reproduced with permission from Chen WP. Asian blepharoplasty. In: Oculoplastic surgery: the essentials. New York: Thieme; 2001:211–24.)

Labels in figure:
- Sub-brow fat (ROOF)
- Orbital septum
- Submuscular fat
- Pretarsal fat

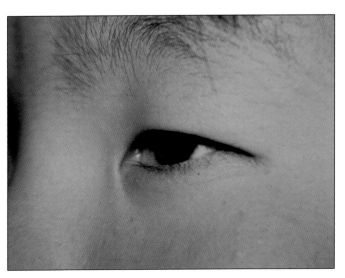

Figure 2.2 Asian upper eyelid with no crease.

Asians, as compared with Americans and Europeans, tend to be more petite. This is simply an observation that their body height, weight, and facial features all tend to be lesser in dimension. The upper tarsal plate (tarsus) of Asians usually measures only in the 6.5 to 8mm range, with the tarsal height in the majority, as measured over the central portion of the upper lid, being within 6.5 to 7.5mm. The upper border of the superior tarsus also corresponds to where a natural upper lid crease would sit, assuming that this is measured in a young adult and that there has not been any involutional change in the lid skin or levator aponeurosis. Compared with a non-Asian's upper tarsus, which is often in the 9–10.5mm range, this is a substantial difference. The critical importance of this clinical observation has to do with the placement of the height (or width as measured from the upper eyelash margin) of the desired crease. If one were to assume that 10 or 11mm is a standard crease and apply it to an Asian face, the resultant look will not be aesthetically acceptable, due to its high placement and proximity to the mid segment of the upper eyelid skin. Other complications, including injury to underlying tissues such as the septum and levator, as well as inadvertent creation of multiple creases and segmentation, may occur.

It has been postulated that Asians without an upper lid crease have a lower point of fusion of the orbital septum onto the anterior surface of the upper tarsus, or that the lower positioning of the preaponeurotic fat pad is the culprit that disrupted or prevented crease formation. It is uncertain as to which came first – whether the anatomically low placement of the orbital septum is the reason for absent crease or the lower migration of the fat. Rather, the true reason may be a lot more and these are just findings by association.

There are at least four types of fat seen in the upper eyelids:

- pretarsal fat;
- preseptal or suborbicularis oculi fat;
- postseptal (preaponeurotic) or orbital fat; and
- submuscular or sub-brow fat.

The preseptal fat of the upper lid and the sub-brow fat seem to occupy contiguous space within the same general tissue plane over the periorbital and suprabrow regions. All four types of fat pads have been observed among Asians with or without an upper lid crease, as well as in Caucasians with crease, thus these four types of fat are not unique to Asians. It is just that among Asians without a crease, the intermingling of these four types of fat seem to be of a greater extent and the boundaries are much less distinct (**Fig. 2.3**).

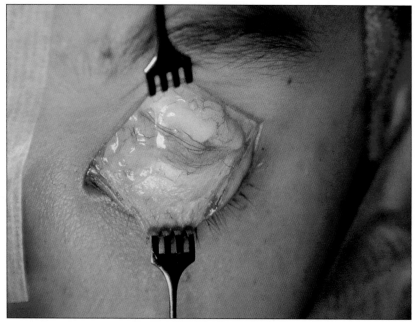

Figure 2.3 Left upper eyelid incision showing three zones of fat pads in this Asian patient: the pure yellowish pretarsal fat pads located in the anterior surface of the upper tarsus and anterior to the opened orbital septum above it; the orange-pinkish vascularized preaponeurotic (postseptal) fat pads with capillaries running horizontally through; and the sub-brow fat pads above the preaponeurotic fat. The sub-brow fat appears pale yellowish, and is located anterior to the opened orbital septum. It may extend inferiorly to become the preseptal fat.

Most Asians have some form of medial canthal folds, even among those who have a crease. The medial canthal fold may be present with the nasally tapered crease (two-thirds to three-quarters of those who have a crease) or with the parallel crease shape. Both are compatible, natural, and not pathologic at all. The majority of requests for medial canthoplasty or epicanthal fold excision are based on preconceived perception or on patients who have pathologic epicanthus associated with congenital blepharophimosis syndrome as reported in the Western medical literature.

Lash ptosis, a secondary downward angulation of the upper eyelashes as a result of the presence of a fold of redundant skin over the ciliary margin, is a feature often seen in Asians without a crease (**Fig. 2.4**). It seldom causes any direct corneal touch or symptoms, and is not to be equated with true trichiasis. Rarely, one does see patients who have corneal touch as a result of prominent eye position, and, even more rare, one may see some Asians who may have very coarse, kinky or straight upper eyelashes, as is sometimes seen in older individuals with the floppy eyelid syndrome.

Epiblepharon is another curious finding sometimes seen in younger Asian patients near the medial portion of their lower eyelids. It may result in secondary trichiasis and can be relieved by simple infraciliary excision of this redundant skin–muscle fold.

Distichiasis, especially medially over the upper as well as the lower lids, may occur and is treated by Asian blepharoplasty of the upper eyelid without any need for tarsal rotation; and in the lower lid by a combination of excision of epiblepharon and/or segmental tarsal rotation.

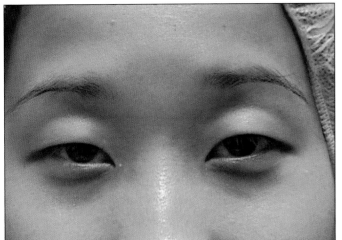

Figure 2.4 Lash ptosis with straight lashes pointing down.

Asians often manifest a subtle head-back position, with the forehead-to-chin plane about 5–10 degrees tilted backwards. Perhaps this is an adaptive head posture to allow greater pupillary clearance with the presence of a single eyelid's redundant fold. We will come back to discuss this point in the section on postoperative management of Asian blepharoplasty patients in Chapter 7.

Curiously, some Asians may manifest a relatively poor upgaze in the absence of clinically noticeable ptosis or known neuromuscular disorders. Some other patients may have only fair or poor levator function; these patients may have true ptosis and this will present a challenge when the time comes to perform ptosis repair as well as attempting to crease a dynamic upper lid crease.

The above two conditions are often associated with an overactive forehead or brow action, as a compensatory move.

The aesthetic purposes of creating an upper lid crease are several fold:

- to enhance and create a visually more apparent eyelid opening, in terms of both the vertical as well as the perceived horizontal dimensions of the palpebral fissure size;

- to create a greater and more consistent platform for the application of cosmetics, eye-shadow, and eyeliners;

- to correct and reverse the downward angulation of the upper eyelashes in patients with absent crease;

- to improve on the vision of those who notice any partial field block or interference in their visual field as a result of the lashes, whether it is secondary trichiasis, or visual awareness of the lashes, which is like seeing through a picket fence when they are downturned;

- to allow freedom from cosmetic application for those who desire it that way; and

- to free the patient from the continued need for application of other non-surgical adjunctive means in order to achieve the goals mentioned above.

Of these, some are aesthetically based and others have a true functional basis.

There are patients who wake up in the morning and spend 30 minutes to 2 hours using Japanese adhesive glue, various adhesive tissue tapes, and even physical manipulations using wires, hairpins, and tooth picks in order to create a temporary crease. Some have been doing it for years and are plainly tired of it.

A nasally tapered crease tends to have a medially converging upper lid crease that may or may not completely join or touch the medial canthal skin (**Fig. 2.5**).

A parallel crease runs parallel across the upper lid margin, still in a concentric fashion to the upper lid margin, but does not converge medially (**Fig. 2.6**).

The crease of a Eurasian may retain one of the two Asian crease shapes but at a wider separation from the lid margin; such subjects often have a more substantial tarsal plate like the parent of the non-Asian side.

Partial crease, segmented crease, and multiple creases (usually no more than two) are further subsets of the ethnic variants and may be seen only in one or in both upper eyelids. It may create asymmetry issues for patients when one side has this condition while the other upper lid is either with or without a crease.

Terminology with respect to Asian lid structures

Commonly, Chinese refer to a nasally tapered crease as an 'inner crease' (converging inward to inner canthus), and the parallel crease as an 'outer crease' ('away' from inner: 'outer' also means to deviate from).

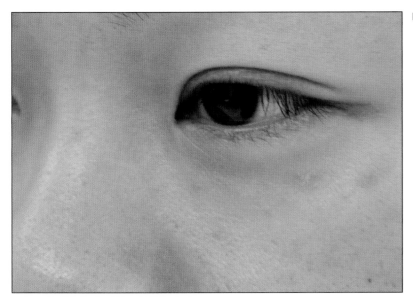

Figure 2.5 Asian upper eyelid with nasally tapered crease.

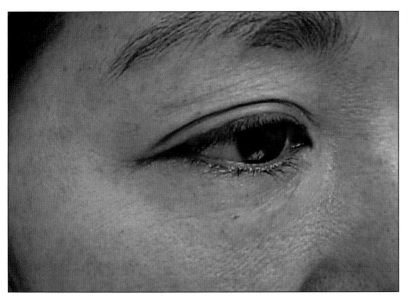

Figure 2.6 Asian upper eyelid with parallel crease.

Anatomy of Upper Eyelid in Caucasians and Non-Asians

The so-called 'Western' or European upper eyelid is distinguished from the 'Asian' upper eyelid by several anatomic differences which produce a 'Western' eyelid crease that is higher and more defined (**Figs 2.7–2.9, Table 2.1**). These differences may reflect several features typical to the 'Western' eyelid:

- absence of pretarsal descent of the preseptal fat pad;

- fusion of the orbital septum with the levator aponeurosis above the tarsal plate;

- a tarsal plate of greater vertical dimension; and

- a lid crease that begins in the medial upper eyelid rather than extending from the medial canthal area.

These eyelid changes correlate broadly with racial phenotypes. Of course, these differences represent generalizations and are only broadly representative rather than specific to individuals of various ethnicities.

The epidermis and dermis of the human eyelid is among the thinnest of the human body and is characterized by loose underlying connective tissue and an absence of subcutaneous fat. It is this combination of an easily engorged layer of loose connective tissue and the impermeable yet highly distensible overlying eyelid skin that permits the exaggerated accumulation of edema that characterizes the postoperative eyelid. The upper eyelid skin is divided into a pretarsal area, a preseptal, and a peri-orbital area. Since the preseptal skin is not anchored to underlying structures, a fold of preseptal skin often overhangs the pretarsal skin and obscures the eyelid crease. The upper eyelid crease is formed by an anterior leaflet of the levator aponeurosis which inserts within the orbicularis oculi. In youth, there is good apposition of the pretarsal eyelid skin to the underlying orbicularis, levator, and tarsus.

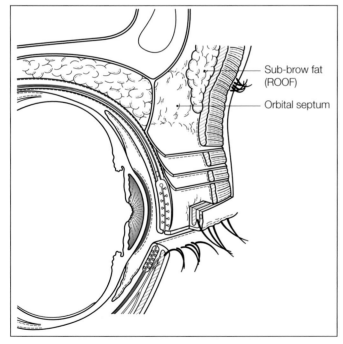

Sub-brow fat (ROOF)

Orbital septum

Figure 2.7 Sagital cross-section of the 'Western' upper eyelid. (Reproduced with permission from Chen WP. Oculoplastic surgery: the essentials. New York: Thieme; 2001:212.)

Table 2.1: Anatomic differences between the 'Western' and 'Asian' eyelid.		
Anatomic feature	**'Western' eyelid**	**'Asian' eyelid**
Preseptal fat pad location	Preseptal	Preseptal and pretarsal
Septum–levator fusion point	Above tarsus	As low as pretarsal plane
Tarsal height	9–10.5mm	6.5–8.0mm
Medial lid crease origin	Medial eyelid	Medial canthus
Presence of crease	100%	50%

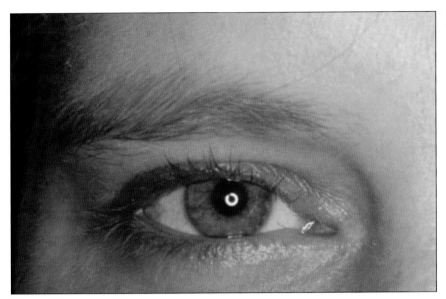

Figure 2.8 The surface features of a youthful 'Western' eyelid.

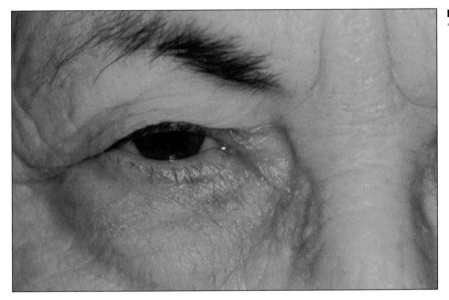

Figure 2.9 The surface features of an aged 'Western' eyelid.

Human eyelid skin

- Epidermis may be only three to four cell layers thick
- Combined epidermis and dermis is less than 1mm thick
- Partially translucent

Deep to the loose subcutaneous connective tissue layer lies the orbicularis oculi muscle (**Fig. 2.10**). The orbicularis oculi serves to close the eyelids and is divided into three contiguous portions: pretarsal, preseptal, and orbital. Each of these layers functions slightly differently, as is demonstrated by their differing origins and insertions. The muscle of Riolan is a specialized portion of the pretarsal orbicularis oculi that corresponds to the gray line and helps to maintain eversion of the eyelashes.

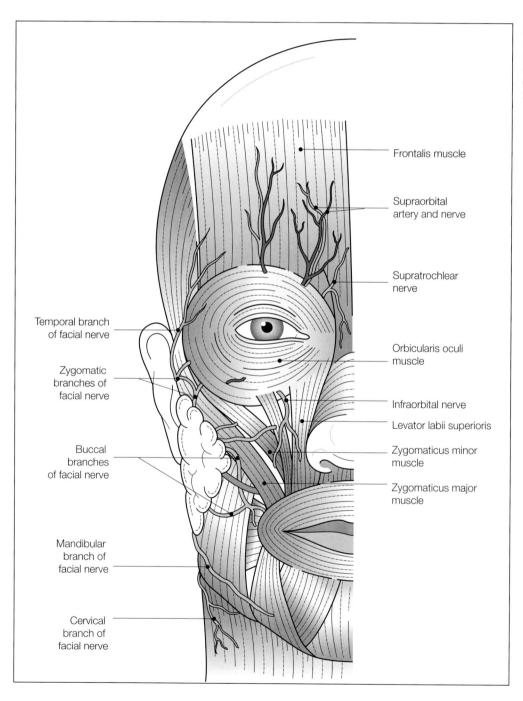

Figure 2.10 The orbicularis oculi and muscles of facial expression. (Reproduced with permission from Chen WP. Oculoplastic surgery: the essentials. New York: Thieme; 2001:5.)

Frontalis muscle

Supraorbital artery and nerve

Supratrochlear nerve

Temporal branch of facial nerve

Orbicularis oculi muscle

Zygomatic branches of facial nerve

Infraorbital nerve

Levator labii superioris

Buccal branches of facial nerve

Zygomaticus minor muscle

Zygomaticus major muscle

Mandibular branch of facial nerve

Cervical branch of facial nerve

Posterior to the orbicularis oculi muscle is the submuscular fascia (also termed the retro-orbicularis fascia and the orbicularis fascia). Running within this well-defined surgical plane are vertically oriented blood vessels and the motor and sensory nerves to the orbicularis and skin. This fascia creates a moderate adherence between the orbicularis and the underlying septum or levator aponeurosis. This fascial plane may be readily divided with strong traction and sharp dissection – thus dividing the eyelid into anterior and posterior lamellae (**Figs 2.11**).

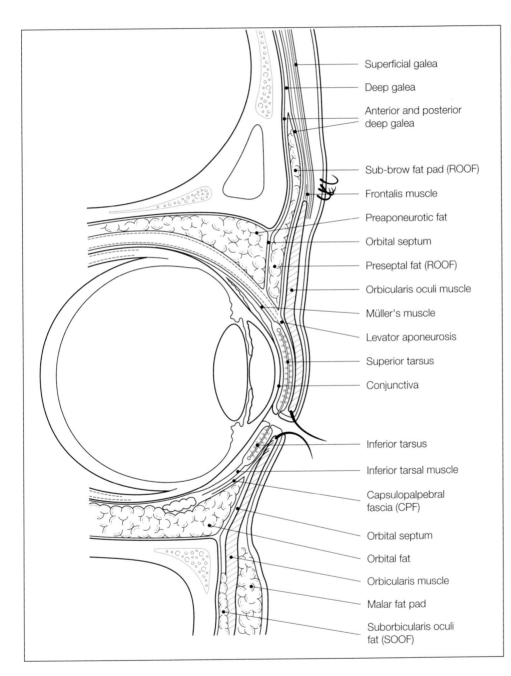

Figure 2.11 Cross-section of upper lid, showing orbital septum, preseptal fat, and preaponeurotic (postseptal) fat. (Reproduced with permission from Chen WP. Oculoplastic surgery: the essentials. New York: Thieme; 2001:4.)

Superficial galea

Deep galea

Anterior and posterior deep galea

Sub-brow fat pad (ROOF)

Frontalis muscle

Preaponeurotic fat

Orbital septum

Preseptal fat (ROOF)

Orbicularis oculi muscle

Müller's muscle

Levator aponeurosis

Superior tarsus

Conjunctiva

Inferior tarsus

Inferior tarsal muscle

Capsulopalpebral fascia (CPF)

Orbital septum

Orbital fat

Orbicularis muscle

Malar fat pad

Suborbicularis oculi fat (SOOF)

The orbital septum (septum orbitale) restrains the central preaponeurotic fat and nasal fat pad of the upper eyelid both anteriorly and inferiorly (**Fig. 2.12**). In the 'Western' upper eyelid, the inferior extent of the orbital septum fuses with the levator aponeurosis at the height of the upper border of the tarsal plate. It is the fusion of these two structures that is believed to limit the inferior descent of the preponeurotic fat pads. Hence, the relatively high point of fusion of the aponeurosis and levator in the 'Western' eyelid contributes to a broader and higher visible pretarsal swath than is seen in the 'Asian' eyelid.

The levator palpebrae superioris is the retractor of the upper eyelid. The distal 14–20mm of aponeurosis is tendinous. The transition from skeletal muscle fibers to glistening white aponeurosis occurs at the level of Whitnall's ligament. After fusing with the orbital septum, the aponeurosis continues inferiorly to insert onto the tarsal plate, pretarsal orbicularis oculi, and pretarsal eyelid skin – thus maintaining apposition of the anterior and posterior eyelid lamella below the eyelid crease. The medial and lateral horns of the levator muscle are attachments towards the medial and lateral canthi.

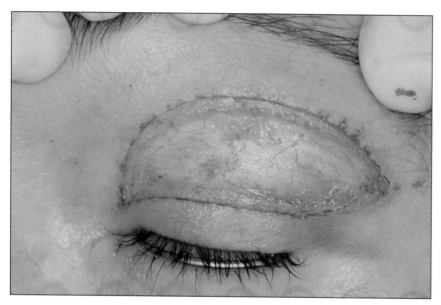

Figure 2.12 This well-defined plane of the orbital septum is revealed following removal of the overlying skin and preseptal orbicularis oculi.

The orbital and palpebral lobes of the lacrimal gland straddle the lateral segment of the levator muscle (**Fig. 2.13**). The tarsal plate of the upper eyelid is 9–10.5mm high and 29mm wide in the 'Western' eyelid. Extending from the lateral commissure to the punctum medially, the tarsus is anchored by the medial and lateral canthal tendons. These three structures form a tarsoligamentous band or sling that helps maintain apposition of the upper eyelid to the globe. The tarsus contains the meibomian glands and their orifices.

Müller's sympathetically innervated smooth muscle arises from the undersurface of the levator palpebrae superioris and descends 15mm to insert on the superior border of the tarsus. Müller's muscle provides 2–3mm of eyelid lift in primary gaze.

Müller's muscle and the tarsus are lined posteriorly by the tarsal and palpebral conjunctiva. The conjunctiva is rich in mucus-secreting goblet cells. Accessory lacrimal glands of Krause and Wolfring reside between the upper tarsal border and the superior fornix. Laterally, the superior fornix is penetrated by the lacrimal gland ductules.

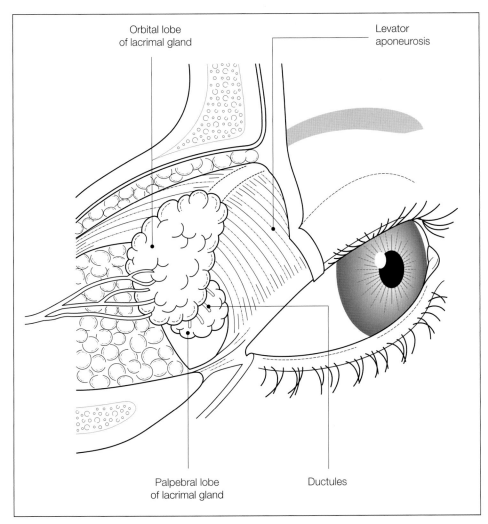

Orbital lobe of lacrimal gland

Levator aponeurosis

Palpebral lobe of lacrimal gland

Ductules

Figure 2.13 Lateral portion of upper lid, showing lacrimal gland. (Reproduced with permission from Chen WP. Oculoplastic surgery: the essentials. New York: Thieme; 2001:17.)

Anatomy of the Lower Lid

Clinically, we do not observe a significant difference between the lower eyelid of Caucasians, Blacks, Hispanics and that of Asians; therefore it will be discussed as one topic. The anatomy of the lower eyelid is very ill defined and is best shown using a series of layered illustrations (**Figs 2.14–2.22**).

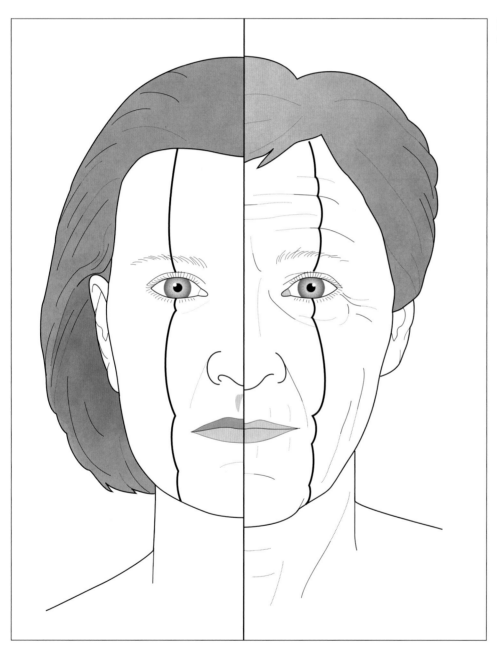

Figure 2.14 The facial changes and cheek laxity that occur with aging.

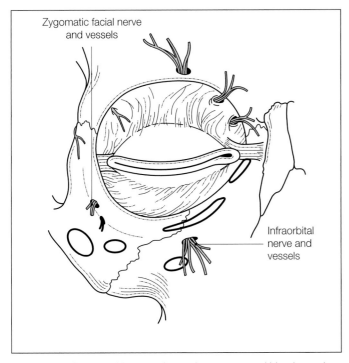

Figure 2.15 The periorbital foraminas, where nerves and blood vessels exit at the deepest plane.

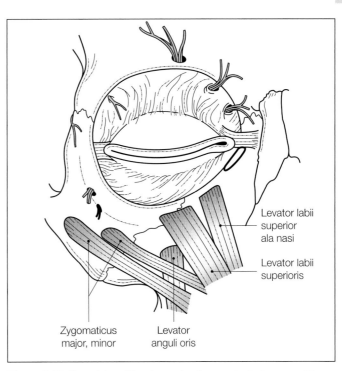

Figure 2.16 The origins of the deep mimetic muscles in the area of the maxilla.

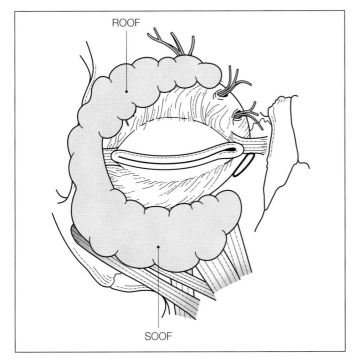

Figure 2.17 The next layer of tissues, which is the suborbicularis oculi fat of the lower eyelid. It extends to the brow and becomes the retro-orbicularis oculi fat (ROOF) under the upper lid.

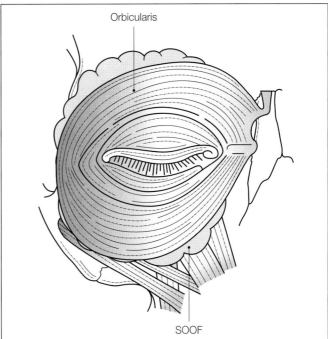

Figure 2.18 The next layer, comprising the pretarsal, preseptal, and periorbital orbicularis oculi muscles. It functions as a closure muscle for the eyelids.

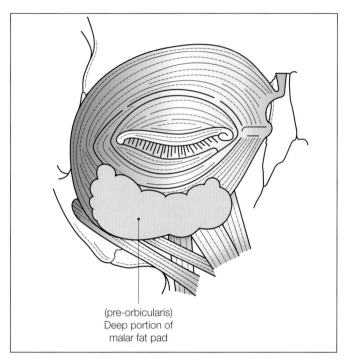

Figure 2.19 The deep portion of the malar fat pads lying over the orbicularis muscles. It is just under and permeated by the superficial musculo-aponeurotic system (SMAS).

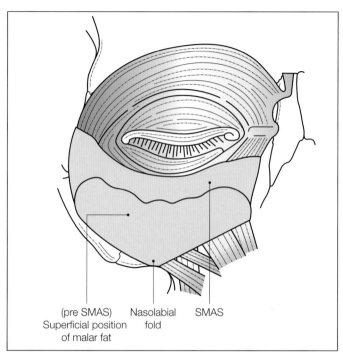

Figure 2.20 The location of the midfacial extent of the superficial musculo-aponeurotic system (SMAS). It lies over the deep portion of the malar fat. The superficial portion of the malar fat lies over the SMAS. The SMAS is blocked inferiorly by the nasolabial fold.

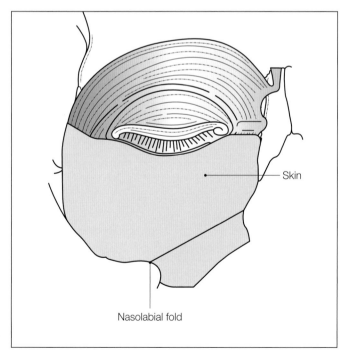

Figure 2.21 Overlying skin and formation of the nasolabial fold.

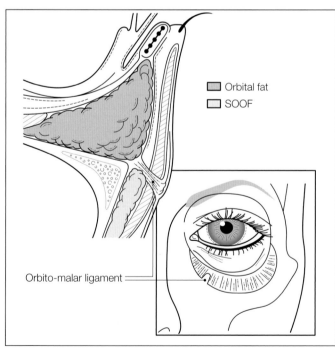

Figure 2.22 The orbital malar ligament. It originates from the orbital rim and combines with (and is considered to be part of) the superficial musculo-aponeurotic system.

Preoperative Preparation, Anesthesia, and Postoperative Considerations

William PD Chen, Jemshed A Khan, and Clinton D McCord Jr

Chapter 3

Preoperative Regimen

For cosmetic blepharoplasty, Dr Chen routinely prescribes 10mg of Valium plus one tablet of Vicodin at 60–90 minutes prior to the procedure. This allows a good period of time for the sedative and analgesic effect to take place. Patients may have been nervous and sleepless the night prior to coming in, or they may have had to travel from a distance, and most will enjoy the relaxation.

About 10 minutes before the scheduled time, he greets his patient and goes through the following check list:

1. Reaffirm the physical findings previously observed and discussed with the patient.
2. Reaffirm the goals of the patient for the surgery that day.
3. Ask if there are any unanswered questions.
4. Take photographs.

The patient is positioned on the operating table in a supine position. A soft foam cushion headrest as well as knee and back support are provided. The nursing staff attach the appropriate monitoring leads, including electrocardiographic, pulse oximetry, as well as grounding pads for monopolar cautery or a radiofrequency transmitter lead.

Intraoperative Regimen

Dr Chen uses 2% Xylocaine with 1:100 000 epinephrine, mixing 10mL with 150 units of hyaluronidase (Wydase), if available*. He then mixes 1mL of the above with 9mL of injectable saline to yield a relatively painless injection (pH balanced, diluted to 0.2% Xylocaine and 1:1 000 000 epinephrine).

*The Pharmacy Services of the New England Compounding Center may offer compounded hyaluronidase. (Telephone 800-994-6322, 697 Waverly Street, Framingham, MA 01702, USA.)

A dose of 0.5mL of 0.2% xylocaine is applied subcutaneously per eyelid. He then waits 2 minutes. Clinical blanching of the skin is observed. Further infiltration of about 0.75–1.5mL of 2% xylocaine (full concentration) per eyelid is then given submuscularly.

A drop of proparacaine is applied per eye for topical anesthesia of the cornea, conjunctiva, and inner surface of the eyelids. The nursing staff prepare the operative field with the appropriate disinfective soap or solutions.

Via a pre-placed butterfly, intravenous aliquots of Versed (midazolam) 0.5mg may be utilized, should further sedation be necessary. Nasal oxygen or room air may be supplied.

Surgical drapes are applied. Dr Chen uses paper drapes as well as an operculated 3M #1020 adhesive drape to minimize any potential gaseous communication between the operative field and the rest of the face under the paper drape. A drop of tetracaine is applied per eye for longer lasting effect.

A black corneo-scleral shell that conforms to the curvature of the cornea and sclera is lubricated with sterile Lacrilube ophthalmic ointment and then applied over the eye to be operated on. The procedure commences.

Ice-cold saline solution is used on the operative field.

In select patients or those who prefer a deeper level of conscious sedation or general anesthesia, the use of an anesthesiologist may be prearranged. This category includes those patients who required cheeklift/midface repositioning, as well as a significant number of those requiring revisions.

Dr Khan's Preoperative Regimen

Most incisional cosmetic procedures are performed in an ambulatory surgery center where monitored anesthesia care is delivered by certified registered nurse anesthetists (CRNA). Patients are greeted and reassured preoperatively and the procedures are confirmed. In the preoperative holding area, supplemental oxygen is provided via nasal cannulae, pulse oximetry and cardiac telemetry are monitored and a heparin lock is placed for intravenous access. In the holding area, patients are rendered amnestic and briefly unconscious with intravenous Versed and Propofol prior to injection with local anesthetic. Usually, the local anesthetic consists of lidocaine 2% with epinephrine 1:100 000 mixed 1:1 with Marcaine 0.75%.

In the operating room, the patient is prepped and then draped with cloth towels. Metal protective eye shields and wet cloth towels are placed if CO_2 laser is to be used. Supplemental oxygen is provided via nasal cannulae, and pulse oximetry, blood pressure monitoring, and cardiac telemetry are continued. Propofol is delivered intraoperatively by the CRNA, if needed. In patients in whom deeper levels of sedation or even unconsciousness are required, supplemental oxygen is delivered to the nasopharynx via a nasal trumpet so as to maintain pO_2 levels despite respiratory depression. This technique allows CO_2 laser resurfacing to be performed without any local anesthetic or endotracheal intubation. Supplemental local anesthetic is often used intraoperatively.

For in-office upper eyelid blepharoplasty, anesthetic discomfort is reduced when each eyelid is pre-injected subcutaneously with 0.75mL solution lidocaine 2% with epinephrine 1:100 000 mixed 1:1 with non-preserved saline. This is followed by an injection of 0.75mL lidocaine 2% with epinephrine 1:100 000. The subcutaneous anesthetic bolus is then milked and manipulated to cover the entire surgical site.

Following surgery, erythromycin ophthalmic ointment may be placed on the eyes or incisions. Patients generally are recovered and discharged within 30 minutes. The eyes and incisions are not usually patched. Stitches (usually 6-0 prolene) are usually removed 9-12 days after surgery.

Postoperative Considerations

The following is a sample of Dr McCord's post-operative instructions:

Scars

Incisions for a blepharoplasty are made in the natural crease of the upper lid, which disguises the final thin scar so that one would have to look very closely in the mirror to determine where an incision had been made, if one can see it at all. In the lower lid, the skin incision is made as close as possible beneath the lash line, and many times extends past the corner of the eye for several millimeters if needed. These incisions leave imperceptible scars. The only area of incision that may be noticeable for a period of time is the outside corner of the eye, in the laugh line area. Some people may require a longer incision or stitch line at the outside corner of the eye in a slightly downsloping direction. This is needed so that the skin may be tensed in the proper way to get good cheekbone definition, and this is true particularly if they have extra folds in the lower cheekbone or mid cheek area. If it is necessary to carry the incision into this area, there usually occurs a small red line, which will fade with time. If one does require an incision above the eyebrow, as will be discussed with the direct brow lift, the incision line is more conspicuous but can be covered with cosmetics until the incision line fades. Although it is unusual to have to do so, dermabrasion can smooth out incision lines that are more conspicuous than one would like, if they do not smooth out on their own. Incisions behind the hairline leave no visible scars and, with the newer techniques, little if any hair loss.

It is important to understand the natural history of healing and scar formation. Tissue glue causes enough healing within a week or ten days such that the incision is strong enough and the stitches can be removed at that time. The incision lines, however, then begin to 'knit'. This process includes the ingrowth of many blood vessels, extracellular material, and other tissue that goes into those areas to strengthen the tissue. During this period of 'knitting' (5–6 weeks), the incision lines will become tight, firm, and reddened, which is the body's response to any cut or incision. This process may not be noticeable to other people but may be noticeable to the patient, and is more a source of frustration than any discomfort. When the body finally recognizes the fact that the tissues are healed enough to suit its purpose

(6–7 weeks), the extra blood vessels and cellular material will leave and the incision lines will soften, bleach, and then fade. The maximum relaxation occurs in about 4 to 5 months. During this period of time – or, for that matter, any time after – it is extremely important to avoid any sunburn or exposure to ultraviolet light in those areas, as this may aggravate and intensify the activity in the incision line.

Stitches

The stitches used are generally nylon stitches or very fine silk sutures, which are removed in 5 to 7 days. Immediately after removal of the stitches, no creams or cosmetics should be used, to avoid tiny cysts that may form along the stitch tracks. About 7–10 days must go by to allow smoothing over of the stitch holes; after this time, one may use cosmetics and cover-up creams, if desired, over the incision lines. Surgical staples or the mini screws associated with the endoscopic eyebrow–forehead lift are usually removed at 10–14 days.

Anesthesia

For the standard eyelid surgery – either upper lids or lower lids by themselves, or upper and lower lids at the same time – usually the surgery can be done with deep sedation (twilight sleep) and local anesthesia that numbs the eyelids. Most people sleep through the procedure. Dr McCord prefers general anesthesia. If one is going to have eyelid surgery combined with the mini-lift of the forehead, or a cheeklift performed with a lower lid blepharoplasty, then a very light 'general' anesthetic is preferred because of the length of the procedure and patient comfort. These procedures can easily be performed on an outpatient basis; however, some people may elect to spend the night after surgery in hospital, for which most hospitals will provide a special rate.

What to expect immediately after surgery

Accentuated appearance

It is normal in the lower lid to have an accentuated tightness in the outside corners, giving an upslant appearance, in the immediate postoperative period and for a while thereafter (usually 3–4 weeks). This

is necessary because of the need to strengthen the lower lid tendon to prevent a pulling down of the lower lid in the swollen period after surgery. This appearance is temporary, but is necessary to prevent the complication of scleral show (excessive white showing under the eye).

Bruising and swelling

There is great variation among individuals with regards to bruising and swelling. It is very rare for a person to get no bruising or swelling at all. Most people will have a puffy and purplish appearance to the eyelids. With the 'standard amount' of bruising and swelling usually seen, most people are presentable for public appearances (with make-up) in 10–14 days.

It is very important for patients to avoid all medications containing aspirin, aspirin-like medications, or any true blood thinners before surgery and for a week after surgery. It is also important to have their blood pressure controlled, in that if the blood pressure is elevated at the time of surgery, they will most certainly bruise more. The most important thing to do to reduce postoperative bruising and swelling is to use ice compresses continuously for the first 48 hours after surgery and as much as possible thereafter. On no occasion should heat compresses be applied to the eyelids during this period. Sometimes, before and after surgery, special medications are given, such as low dose cortisone, to help prevent the tissue reacting so much to the surgery.

Eye lubrication and blurred vision

Our main concern for the health of the eye is the prevention of 'dry spots' that can occur after surgery. Because there will be some 'tightness' of the eyelids following surgery, we require the patient to apply lubricants to his or her eyes, particularly at nighttime, to avoid any dryness or symptoms of dryness. All tear production is examined before surgery; however, in some rare situations, a person may be required to use lubricating drops after surgery to allow his or her eyes to be comfortable. Immediately after surgery, we prefer the use of ointments, which are much more effective at preventing dry spots; however, most people do not like them because they do blur the vision. This extra lubrication is needed right after the operation for protection of the eye from dry spots and chemosis. To reduce postoperative chemosis, we apply a 6.0 nylon tarsorrhaphy suture through the upper and lower tarsal plates 1mm lateral to temporal limbus prior to completion of the case. After the stitches are removed, one can, in most cases, switch to artificial teardrops, which do not blur the vision.

Physical activity

The first 2 days are completely devoted to ice compresses and head elevation and remaining quiet. Walking around and sedentary activity can take place following the first 2 days until suture removal. The ice compresses can be used intermittently during this period (usually 30 minutes, four to five times a day). It would be possible to drive a car during this period if there was a definite need; however, the vision will be very blurred from the use of the ointment and the stiffness of the eyelids. There should be no exercise (aerobics, jogging, etc.) the first week. In the second week, no exercise should occur that places a strain on the incisions; however, some walking and stretching can be done.

Only after the first 2 weeks should exercise that raises the heart rate be undertaken. The 'extra blood' that may be pumped through the operated area might cause swelling. If this occurs, then the patient should stop and apply ice to the area.

Common patient worries

The two things that generally concern people the most immediately after surgery are:

- body image; and
- blurred vision.

Body image Most people have a puffy and purplish look to their eyelids immediately after surgery. There will also be the overly tight or very tense look in the corners of their eyes if they have had lower lid surgery. This appearance can cause initial 'patient remorse' since they may not have seen themselves with this appearance unless they have had previous surgery. This is, of course, the normal appearance following this type of surgery, and, with time, the puffiness and bruising will go away and their eyelid contours will resume to the desired appearance.

Blurred vision Immediately after surgery, the patients' vision will be blurred to the point that they will not be able to read very well. The reasons are that their eyelids, which are basically windshield wipers, will be stiff for a period of time and will not be able to wipe (their cornea) properly. Also, they will be using lubricating ointment in their eyes to prevent dry spots, which will add to the blurring.

It is very important that the patient's family or those who will be caring for the patient after surgery know and expect these changes so they will not have concern.

Safety With Blepharoplasty Surgery

Our goal is to try to have the happiest patient possible following surgery, with the best possible improvement in the person's appearance, but not at the expense of eye safety. The eyelids are not decorations and their purpose is to protect the eye. They must function properly following any eyelid surgery. There is always some stiffness after eyelid surgery of this type, which may persist for a while; however, patients who have good eye moisture and good eye movements usually do fine. Many patients do use some artificial teardrops after surgery. Our approach is to be safe and conservative in the amount of skin that is removed. If there are some residual folds after healing (not quite enough skin taken), they can easily be trimmed later in the office. If too much skin is removed, it is not an easy situation to rectify, as this may require skin recruitment from elsewhere.

Secondary Surgery or 'Touch-up' Surgery

For primary patients who require secondary or 'touch-up' surgery, if it seems appropriate, there is no surgical charge, but medical supplies (stitches, etc.) are charged for. If it is established that there is no contraindication, residual folds can be removed, or, if needed, adjustment of the lower lid can be done. The most common touch-up is removal of folds of skin in the upper lid at the outside corner just under the brow, or adjustment of the outside corner of the lower lid. If the adjustment is more than minor, it must be done on an outpatient basis at a surgical facility.

Complications of Surgery

Fortunately, there are few true complications – most of the postoperative concerns are whether or not to do any 'touch-up' work – however, it is important to discuss here some of the complications associated with any eyelid surgery. A very serious complication would be some unfavorable reaction to the anesthetic medicine, either the local or the other agents that are used. Eyelid complications, as mentioned before, are usually a lower lid pull down or out turning following surgery, owing to shrinkage of skin or excessive skin removal in that area. This is much more of a risk in people who have extremely lax lower lids and can be aggravated if, in addition, the person has serious bruising or hematoma formation. In such people, additional tightening of the ligaments in the lower lid is deemed necessary to prevent this complication. Other possible complications include infection and hemorrhage.

Insurance Claims and Office Policy

Patients should not expect any insurance company to pay the surgical fee for surgery that may be considered cosmetic or medically unnecessary in nature. If patients feel that they would like to involve their insurance company, they are strongly advised to attempt to get a 'prior approval' from such. Unfortunately, many insurance companies will only give equivocal statements regarding possible future coverage of surgery. If, in the 'prior approval', the insurance company indicates a specific amount they will pay for the surgery, then that amount will be subtracted from the patient's presurgical deposit. If the insurance company will not commit to a definite amount, then the patient will be responsible for the full surgical deposit, and, after surgery, any amount the insurance pays will be reimbursed to the patient.

Other Interested Parties

As mentioned previously, in many cases a spouse or close friend will be involved in a patient's postoperative care and observe the patient in his or her postoperative course. If they have not had the opportunity to make the preoperative consultation visits with the patient, they will be unfamiliar with the usual side effects of surgery and what is normal after surgery. For their awareness, they should read the information sheets provided. In most cases, it may be appropriate for them to see the preoperative videos in the office or have consultation with the surgeon before surgery, for better understanding of blepharoplasty surgery and its possible postoperative side effects.

Endoscopic-assisted Eyebrow Surgery

Clinton D McCord Jr

The upper lid and the eyebrow behave as a unit and are interdependent. Commonly, eyebrow procedures are needed for stabilization before performing the upper lid blepharoplasty. Because of this sequence, the eyebrow procedures are discussed first.

Normally, eyebrows are positioned above the level of the superior orbital rim, but, with age, may migrate below the rim, causing redundancy and folding of the upper eyelid skin. This process also produces a narrowed spacing between the eyebrow hairs and the lashes, which can cause a frowning appearance in the patient. The mechanics of brow ptosis are similar to those of a curtain rod that has loosened and fallen, causing folding in the curtain.

It is important to recognize the problem of eyebrow laxity before performing upper lid blepharoplasty, because failure to correct brow laxity or displacement before the blepharoplasty will impair the result.

The aim of upper lid blepharoplasty is to remove redundant skinfolds and produce a clear strip of skin above the eyelash line (the eye-shadow space in females). In order for the surgeon to achieve this, any pre-existing laxity or ptosis of the eyebrows must be surgically corrected. Eyebrow procedures, in most cases, must be performed before the blepharoplasty procedure.

Anatomy

It is important to have firm knowledge of anatomy in the eyebrow area to avoid complications and to produce the best possible result with eyebrow surgery. Appreciation of the anatomic relationship of the frontal branch of the facial nerve to the fascial layers is important to define the safe level of dissection for protecting the nerve when operating in the brow and temporal region.

Fascia and attachments

There are three fascial layers in the temporal region that are important landmarks for localization of the frontal branch of the facial nerve. The superficial temporal fascia is the most superficial layer. The deep temporal fascia is made up of a superficial layer and a deep layer (**Fig. 4.1**).

The *deep temporal fascia* is a dense double-layered fascia covering the temporalis muscle. The temporal line of fusion is a transverse line at the level of the superior orbital rim, extending laterally over the fascia, and represents fusion of the two layers superior to this line. The fascia is separated inferior to the line by the superficial temporal fat pad, which is located between the superficial and deep layers of the deep temporal fascia and extends to the level of the zygomatic arch. The deep temporal fat pad lies beneath the deep temporal fascia 2cm above the zygomatic arch and overlies the temporalis muscle and tendon; it is an extension of the buccal fat pad through the zygomatic arch.

The *superficial temporal fascia* is the layer that contains the frontal branch of the facial nerve on its deep subaponeurotic surface. This layer represents an extension of the submuscular aponeurotic system (SMAS). The subaponeurotic plane consists of loose areolar tissue that separates the superficial temporal fascia from the deep temporal fascia. The subaponeurotic plane is avascular and extends inferiorly to the zygomatic arch. The temporal region of the subaponeurotic space and the subperiosteal space are connected by division of the periosteal reflection along the superior temporal line that marks the origin of the deep temporal fascia. This transition zone lies along the anterior crest of the temporal bone.

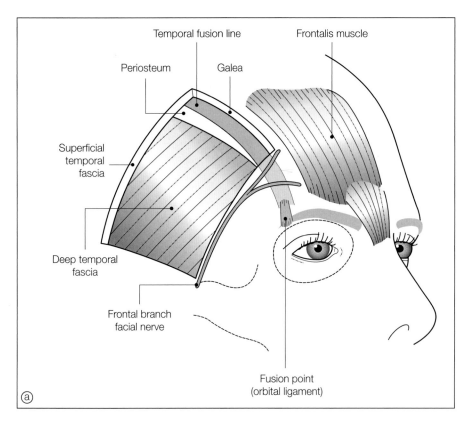

Temporal fusion line

Frontalis muscle

Periosteum

Galea

Superficial temporal fascia

Deep temporal fascia

Frontal branch facial nerve

Fusion point (orbital ligament)

(a)

Figure 4.1 (a) The fascial and muscular planes in the scalp and forehead area. The course of the frontal branch of the facial nerve is shown traveling through the superficial temporal fascia. (Reproduced with permission from Chen WP. Oculoplastic surgery: the essentials. New York: Thieme; 2001: 127.)

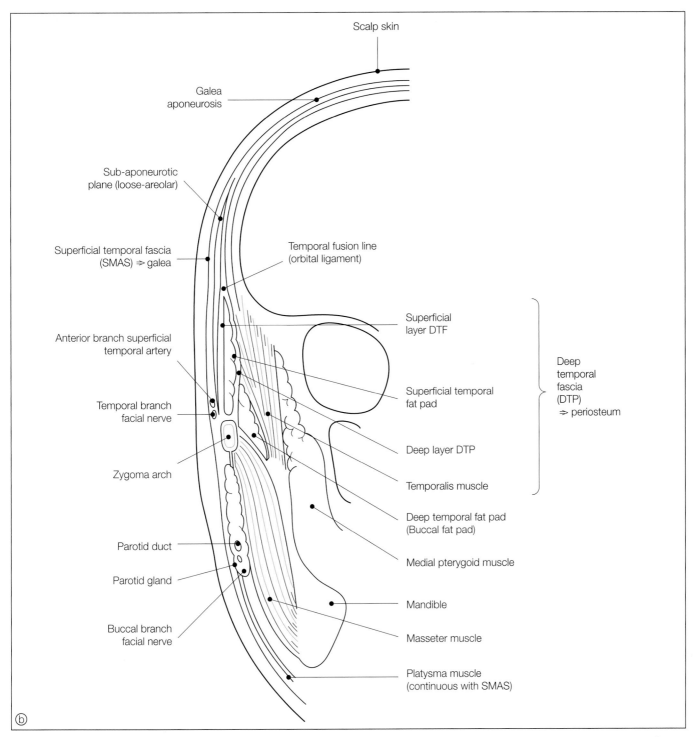

Scalp skin

Galea aponeurosis

Sub-aponeurotic plane (loose-areolar)

Superficial temporal fascia (SMAS) ⇒ galea

Temporal fusion line (orbital ligament)

Anterior branch superficial temporal artery

Superficial layer DTF

Superficial temporal fat pad

Deep temporal fascia (DTP) ⇒ periosteum

Temporal branch facial nerve

Deep layer DTP

Zygoma arch

Temporalis muscle

Deep temporal fat pad (Buccal fat pad)

Medial pterygoid muscle

Parotid duct

Parotid gland

Mandible

Masseter muscle

Buccal branch facial nerve

Platysma muscle (continuous with SMAS)

(b)

Figure 4.1 (b) On the temporal side of the face, the galea aponeurosis covers the fascia of the temporalis muscle as the superficial temporal fascia (SMAS, superficial musculo-aponeurotic system). Just superior to the zygomatic arch, the temporal branch of the facial nerve and the anterior branch of the superficial temporal artery lie within this plane of the SMAS. The galea splits into the superficial and deep temporal fasciae (DTF) at the superior origin of the temporalis muscle on the skull. Further inferiorly, at the line of fusion, the deep temporal fascia splits into a superficial and a deep layer, with both attaching to the zygoma. The superficial temporal fat pad lies deep to the superficial layer of the DTF, whereas the deep temporal fat pad beneath the deep layer of the DTF is a superior extension for the buccal fat pad. Below the zygoma, the parotid gland lies between the SMAS and the masseter muscle. Further inferiorly, the SMAS is contiguous with the platysma muscle. The masticatory muscles of the temporalis and medial pterygoid insert onto the medial side of the mandible, whereas the masseter inserts onto the lateral side. (Reproduced with permission from Chen WP. Oculoplastic surgery: the essentials. New York: Thieme; 2001: 127.)

The galea is contiguous with the superficial temporal fascia, and the periosteum of the skull is continuous with the deep temporal fascia. The confluence of these fascial planes to the skull and attachment to the brow tissue have a characteristic configuration known as the fusion line and orbital ligament. This confluence produces a vertical band 5–6mm wide just medial to the temporal fusion line of the skull, which has a continuation as the superior temporal line. In this area, the deep layers of the superficial temporal fascia and the galea are bonded to the periosteum and fixed to the bone (**Fig. 4.2**). At the edge of the orbital rim in this fusion line is a fibrous band attached to the bone, called the orbital ligament, which can limit superficial temporal fascia movement and effectively tethers the lateral eyebrow to the orbital rim.

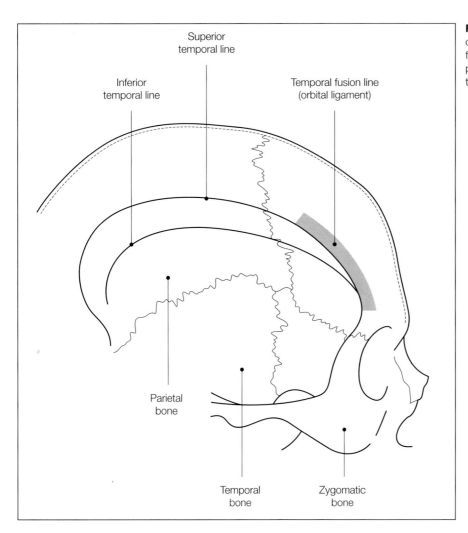

Superior
temporal line

Inferior
temporal line

Temporal fusion line
(orbital ligament)

Parietal
bone

Temporal
bone

Zygomatic
bone

Figure 4.2 The insertion lines of the fascia planes on the skull in the placement of the temporal fusion line and orbital ligament. (Reproduced with permission from Chen WP. Oculoplastic surgery: the essentials. New York: Thieme; 2001: 127.)

Motor and sensory nerves

The frontal branch of the facial nerve provides motor innervation to the frontalis and corrugator muscles. The course and depth of the nerve has been well defined and extends along a line beginning 0.5cm below the tragus to 1.5cm above the lateral aspect of the brow.

The frontal branch lies within the superficial temporal fascia as it traverses the zygomatic arch, and is at greatest risk for injury at this level.

Superior to the zygomatic arch, the nerve is superficial to the superficial layer of the deep temporal fascia, within the superficial temporal fascia.

The supratrochlear and supraorbital nerves provide sensory innervation to the scalp, forehead, and eyelid region. The ophthalmic (V_1) division of the trigeminal nerve traverses the cavenous sinus and enters the orbit through the superior orbital fissure. The ophthalmic nerve has three divisions: frontal, nasociliary, and lacrimal. The frontal nerve runs along the superior aspect of the orbit and divides into the supratrochlear and supraorbital nerves. The supratrochlear nerve emerges from the medial aspect of the superior orbital rim and provides sensory innervation to the glabella, medial forehead, medial upper eyelid, and conjunctiva. The supraorbital nerve exits the orbit in the central aspect of the superior orbital rim most commonly through a notch. A true supraorbital foramen exists as an anatomic variant in 25% of orbits. The supraorbital nerve provides sensory innervation to the scalp, lateral forehead, lateral upper eyelid, and conjunctiva.

Muscles of animation

The musculature in the forehead and brow that contributes to animation in the forehead and glabella region includes the frontalis, procerus, and corrugator supercilii muscles (**Fig. 4.3**).

The frontalis muscle travels above the galea and is the elevator of the eyebrow and glabella area. Its insertion does not extend past the fusion line and has reduced effect in the lateral brow. It is a paired muscle that is an extension of the galea aponeurotica and occipitalis muscle. The vertically oriented fibers insert into the supraorbital dermis and elevate the eyebrow during contraction. Increased frontalis activity, which is needed to maintain an elevated brow position in response to brow ptosis, can cause transverse lines across the forehead. The frontalis muscle is a primary brow elevator and should therefore not be weakened during a procedure aimed at brow elevation.

The procerus muscle is a midline muscle that originates from the nasal bones and upper lateral cartilages. The vertically oriented fibers insert into the dermis of the glabella at the medial border of the frontalis. Contraction of the procerus causes inferior and medial displacement of the medial eyebrow and a transverse line at the nasal radix. The procerus muscle has innervation from the buccal branch of the facial nerve. The procerus is a primary brow depressor and therefore should be weakened to achieve medial brow elevation.

The corrugator supercilii muscle is a paired muscle that originates from the periosteum of the superior medial orbital rim. The fibers are oriented in an oblique direction, inserting into the dermis of the medial eyebrow skin with lateral interdigitations with the medial portion of the orbicularis oculi muscle. Contraction of the corrugator muscles causes inferior and medial displacement of the eyebrow and the vertical oblique lines of the glabella. Weakening the medial portion of the corrugator contributes to medial brow elevation and correction of glabellar frown lines. The lateral portion of the corrugator is felt to produce slight lateral brow elevation and should be preserved. Motor innervation of the corrugator is from the frontal branch of the facial nerve.

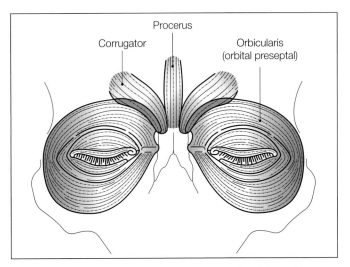

Figure 4.3 The protractor muscles of the brow and eyelid area. The corrugator and procerus muscles together with a portion of orbicularis nasally are brow depressors. Laterally, orbicularis fibers act as depressors of the tail of the brow. (Reproduced with permission from Chen WP. Oculoplastic surgery: the essentials. New York: Thieme; 2001: 128.)

Changes in the Eyebrow with Age

The development of eyebrow laxity and ptosis with aging is attributed to the progressive laxity of the scalp and forehead soft tissues over time. This mechanism, aided by gravity, can produce an overall symmetrical downward displacement of the eyebrow with narrowing of the spacing between the eyebrows and eyelashes (decreased brow–lash distance). There are specific forces and tissue conditions in the lateral and nasal eyebrow that may allow selective depression of those areas. In the lateral portion or tail of the eyebrow, the force of orbicularis contracture, and increased mobility, allowed by fatty layers in the area, are added to the forces of gravity and laxity, causing more selective brow ptosis in that area. In the nasal portion of the brow, the depressor muscles, corrugator supraciliaris, and procerus, together with contracture of some local orbicularis fibers, serve to counteract the lifting effect of the frontalis muscle and bring the nasal brow downward (**Fig. 4.4**). The shape of the eyebrow is usually more arched in females and flatter in males, and may remain so with age.

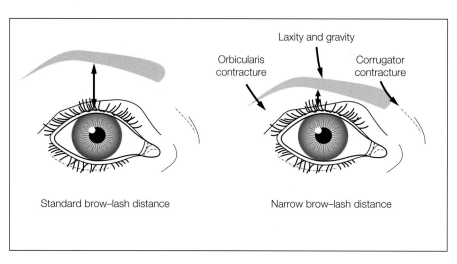

Figure 4.4 The normal brow spacing and position (left) and the downward displacement of the brow from forces counteracting the frontalis muscle elevation (right). (Reproduced with permission from Chen WP. Oculoplastic surgery: the essentials. New York: Thieme; 2001: 131.)

Endoscopic-assisted Eyebrow Forehead Lift

In recent years, it has been more common to perform the eyebrow forehead lift with endoscopic assistance through small incisions. I use this procedure primarily in females for correction of ptosis in the nasal two-thirds of the brow and the frowning contracture lines in the glabellar area. I also use this procedure, usually supplemented with an internal browpexy performed through an upper blepharoplasty incision, to correct ptosis or laxity in the lateral third of the brow.

Surgical technique and instrumentation

Instrumentation includes a camera and video equipment, endoscope, light source, retractor, and endoscopic surgical instruments (graspers and periosteal elevators with varying curves). These instruments are used to create the subperiosteal optical space, in which the procedure is performed. The development of this space is the primary requirement in endoscopic surgery, and visibility is maintained by a retractor-mounted endoscopic system (**Fig. 4.5**).

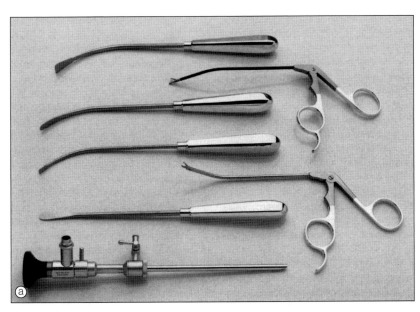

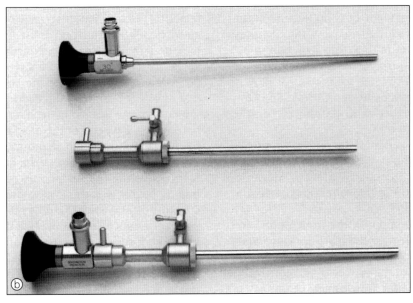

Figure 4.5 Endoscopic system and instrumentations. (a) Variety of periosteal elevators, insulated grasper, insulated scissors and endoscope in irrigating sleeve. (b) Endoscope and detached irrigating sleeve, and endoscope in irrigating sleeve. (Instruments courtesy of Snowdon Pencer.) (Reproduced with permission from McCord CD. Eyelid surgery: principles and techniques. Philadelphia: Lippincott-Raven; 1995: 369.)

Various camera systems include one-chip, three-chip, and digital formats. The video cart setup generally includes a high-resolution video monitor, VCR and printer, camera source, and a light source with fiberoptic attachment to the endoscope. The currently available endoscopes are rigid, glass, Hopkins rod-type endoscopes. Because the size of the optical cavity that can be created during endoscopic brow lift is limited, the 5mm external diameter endoscope size is recommended. Various angles of visualization with the endoscope are available, but the 30-degree downward view is most commonly used to view the anatomy in the supraorbital region. The optical cavity is maintained through tissue retraction using the retractor-mounted endoscopic system or with the use of a special sleeve or spoon that extends beyond the end of the endoscope (**Fig. 4.6**).

The patient is placed on the operating table with the head extended slightly beyond the headrest, to facilitate clearance for the use of the endoscope and instruments. The procedure is usually performed under general anesthesia. Generous infiltration with 0.25% Xylocaine with epinephrine (1:400 000) is used in the scalp and forehead area for hemostasis (**Fig. 4.7**).

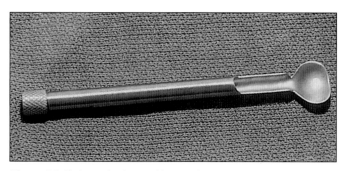

Figure 4.6 Endoscopic sleeve with retracting spoon extension. (Reproduced with permission from Chen WP. Oculoplastic surgery: the essentials. New York: Thieme; 2001: 131.)

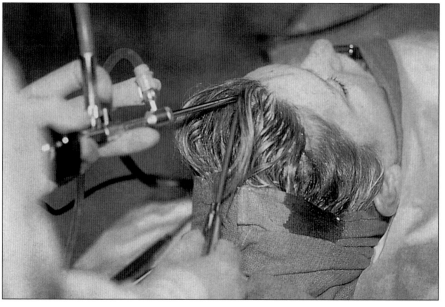

Figure 4.7 Operating room set-up and orientation of surgeon to patient. (Reproduced with permission from Chen WP. Oculoplastic surgery: the essentials. New York: Thieme; 2001: 133.)

Placement of scalp incisions

Three scalp incisions are made – one midline and two lateral (**Fig. 4.8**). The location of the lateral incisions depends on the desired vector of pull on the eyebrow. In patients who have unusually severe nasal brow laxity and glabellar folding, the incisions are placed closer to the midline incision, to gain maximum traction, and closer to the nasal brow and glabellar area. In patients with general brow laxity, the lateral incisions are placed in a wider pattern and slanted to produce both nasal and some temporal elevation. All incisions are placed behind the hairline to minimize scar visibility. If possible, incisions should avoid sites of maximal hairline recession.

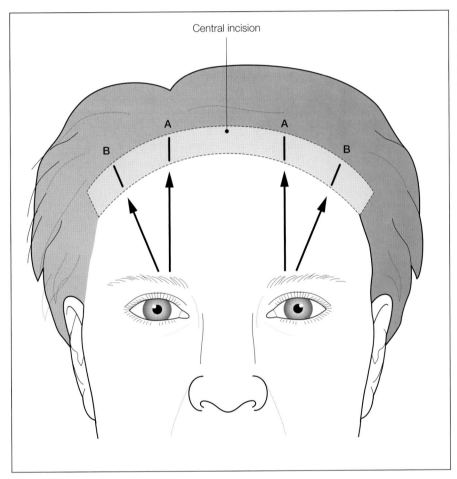

Figure 4.8 Placement of three incisions for endoscopic-assisted eyebrow forehead lift. The central incision serves as a port for the endoscope. The lateral incisions serve only as openings for placement of screw fixation. Position A for the lateral incisions is used for patients who require maximum nasal brow and glabellar lift. Position B is for patients who need more general brow elevation. (Reproduced with permission from Chen WP. Oculoplastic surgery: the essentials. New York: Thieme; 2001: 131.)

Creation of an optical space

The initial optical space is created with a subperiosteal dissection using a straight elevator through the three scalp incisions. Undermining in the subperiosteal space extends initially to within 1cm of the supraorbital rim and to the superior temporal line laterally. Undermining behind the scalp incisions is also performed to prevent redundancy and folding when the forehead and scalp are advanced posteriorly (**Fig. 4.9**). The subperiosteal plane has an advantage of firm postoperative reattachment with healing following brow elevation. Initially, subperiosteal dissection is begun anteriorly through the central incision without using the endoscope, stopping 1–2cm above the superior orbital rim.

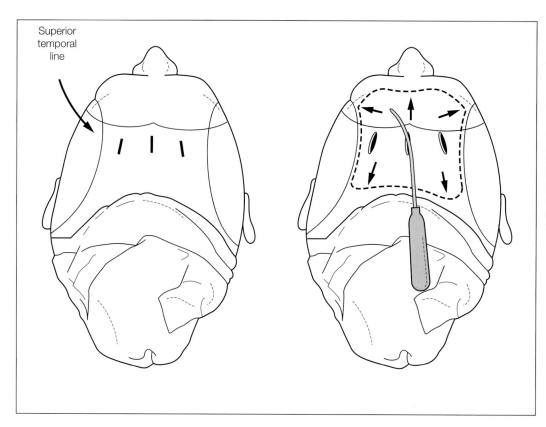

Superior temporal line

Figure 4.9 Left: Placement of three incisions for endoscopic-assisted eyebrow forehead lift. The central incision serves as a port for the endoscope. The lateral incisions serve only as openings for placement of screw fixation. Right: The area of periosteal undermining performed for visualization before the endoscope is inserted. (Reproduced with permission from Chen WP. Oculoplastic surgery: the essentials. New York: Thieme; 2001: 132.)

At this point, the endoscope with a retraction sleeve and spoon is inserted through the central incision into the optical cavity to continue subperiosteal dissection in the lower forehead under endoscopic visualization. The dissection then proceeds down to the superior orbital rim with direct visualization (**Fig. 4.10**). Several different sizes and curves of periosteal elevators are available for use, depending on the contour of the frontal bone and the distance from the brow to the hairline.

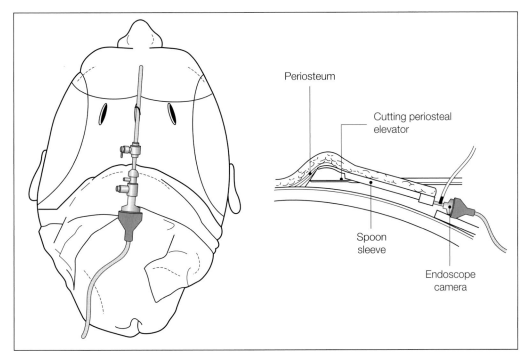

Periosteum

Cutting periosteal elevator

Spoon sleeve

Endoscope camera

Figure 4.10 Insertion of the endoscope with retracting spoon through the central incision and the insertion of a periosteal elevator (or other endoscopic tool) through a lateral incision (left). The spoon extension on the endoscope allows better retraction of the brow tissue for visualization (right).
(Reproduced with permission from Chen WP. Oculoplastic surgery: the essentials. New York: Thieme; 2001: 132.)

Periosteal release

Once adequate visualization of the optical cavity to the orbital rim has been achieved, the surgeon places a horizontal relaxing incision through the periosteum. The periosteum is divided along the edge of the supraorbital rim transversely with a relaxing incision using a sharp periosteal elevator (**Fig. 4.11**). A curved periosteal hook or curved endoscopic scissors can be used to divide the periosteum. Periosteal division continues laterally along the orbital rim to the level of the lateral canthus using a narrow, curved elevator. The procerus and corrugator muscles can then be visualized centrally once the periosteum is divided.

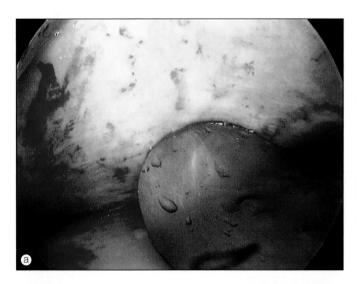

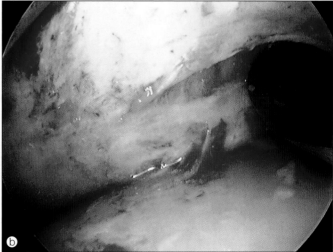

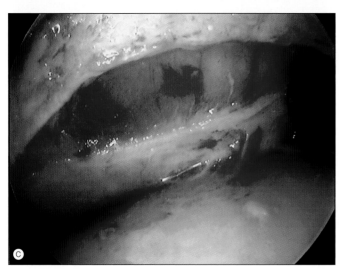

Figure 4.11 Intraoperative endoscopic images showing creation of relaxing incision through the periosteum at the level of the superior orbital rim. (a) Insertion of reversed sharp periosteal elevator to the periosteum. Initial periosteal incision (b) and extension laterally (c). (Reproduced with permission from Chen WP. Oculoplastic surgery: the essentials. New York: Thieme; 2001: 133.)

Resection of corrugator and procerus muscles

Once the opening of the periosteum has been completed, biopsy forceps are introduced and used to resect portions of the procerus and corrugator muscles that cause the glabellar frown lines. Hypertrophy of the procerus or corrugator muscles produced by repeated frowning is improved by the myectomy, which weakens these muscles. A variety of biopsy forceps are available; however, blunt-tipped Takahashi biopsy forceps allow precise muscle resection, which minimizes the potential overdissection of the underlying subcutaneous tissue and dermis, which could result in a visible deformity in the glabellar region. Removal of the procerus is first performed in the midline at the level of the superior orbital rim. Dissection then proceeds laterally, with removal of the corrugator on both sides of the supratrochlear nerve (**Fig. 4.12**). The supratrochlear nerve crosses the corrugator and is deep to the orbicularis oculi fibers. A nerve hook can be used to retract the supratrochlear nerve. The supratrochlear nerves can be seen with the underlying oblique fibers of the corrugator muscle and the transverse supratrochlear vein.

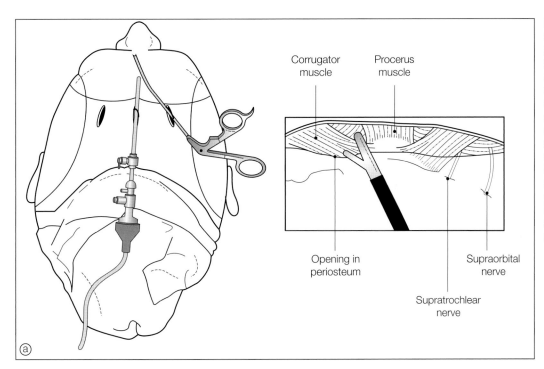

Corrugator muscle

Procerus muscle

Opening in periosteum

Supratrochlear nerve

Supraorbital nerve

ⓐ

Figure 4.12 (a) Insertion through the opening in the periosteum of a grasping device for partial resection of corrugator and procerus muscles. Branches of the supratrochlear nerve are contained within the corrugator and should be spared. The supraorbital nerve is usually visualized laterally in the notch but is away from the resection area. (Reproduced with permission from Chen WP. Oculoplastic surgery: the essentials. New York: Thieme; 2001: 134.)

The supraorbital nerves are visualized laterally. Following procerus and corrugator myectomy, inspection for hemostasis is performed. Electrocautery using an insulated grasper controls any bleeding points.

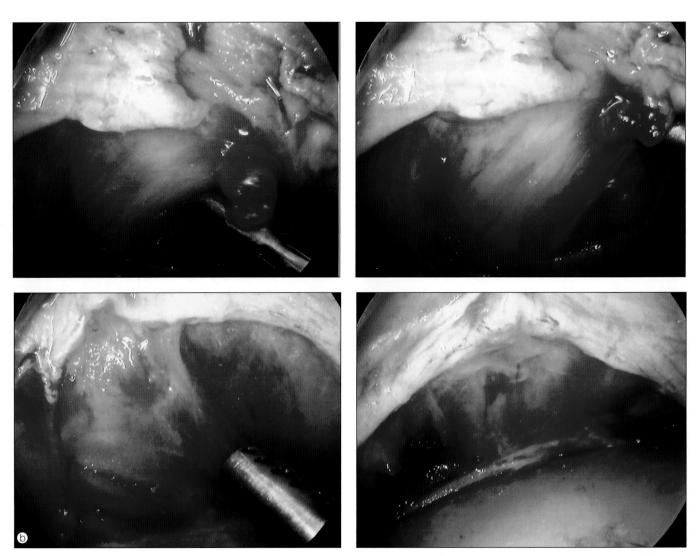

Figure 4.12 (b) Endoscopic images showing excision of corrugator muscles. Top left and right: Stripping of the corrugator on the right side utilizing a Takahashi biopsy forceps. Bottom left: Forceps pointing at left corrugator, with portion of supratrochlear nerve visible within the muscle. Bottom right: View of glabellar area after corrugators have been stripped bilaterally.

Brow and forehead elevation and fixation

The forehead and scalp are then advanced upward and retracted to produce brow elevation so that fixation of the tissue can be performed. Several methods of fixation have been used. This author favors the screw fixation methods. Screw fixation methods have included the permanent placement of surgical screws that anchor galeal support sutures or are temporary percutaneous screws that are removed 1 to 2 weeks after surgery and rely on periosteal adhesions for permanency. Only the lateral incisions are used for fixation. A guarded drill bit 4mm in depth (**Fig. 4.13**) is used to place a drill hole in the calvarium at the posterior edge of the lateral incisions. There is some repositioning of the lateral incisions posteriorly by traction before the drill holes are made. A 2mm-diameter titanium screw, 12mm in length, is then placed in the hole, thereby allowing an 8mm length to traverse the scalp so that the screw head remains external to the scalp (**Fig. 4.14**).

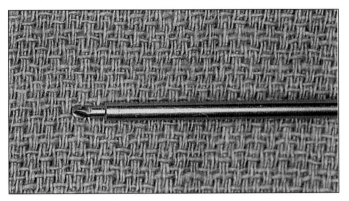

Figure 4.13 A drill bit with a 4mm guard used to create drill holes in the calvarium at the posterior edges of the lateral scalp incisions. (Reproduced with permission from Chen WP. Oculoplastic surgery: the essentials. New York: Thieme; 2001: 135.)

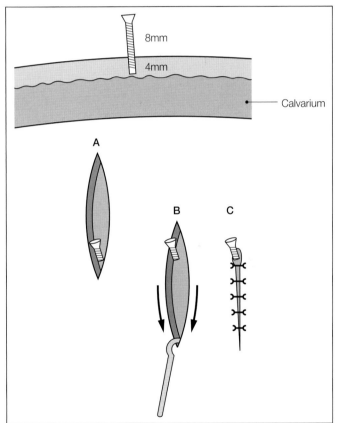

Figure 4.14 Placement of screw in the calvarium at the posterior edge of a lateral incision. (Reproduced with permission from Chen WP. Oculoplastic surgery: the essentials. New York: Thieme; 2001: 135.)

Once the screw is secured at the posterior aspect of the lateral radial incisions (**Fig. 4.15**), the scalp is advanced posteriorly along the vector of the incision with a single-hook retractor (**Fig. 4.16**).

After the scalp has been advanced to achieve proper brow elevation with some consideration for overcorrection, surgical staples are placed posterior to the screw to close the incision and maintain the scalp advancement (**Fig. 4.17**). All remaining scalp incisions are closed with staples.

Staple and screw removal occurs 10 to 14 days after surgery. No drains are required. The postoperative edema is mild and the incidence of hematoma is low.

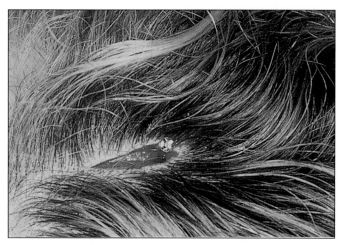

Figure 4.15 Positioning of the 12mm screw in the calvarium. (Reproduced with permission from Chen WP. Oculoplastic surgery: the essentials. New York: Thieme; 2001: 135.)

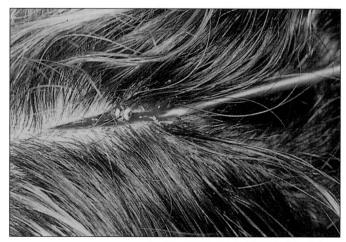

Figure 4.16 Retraction of scalp with large skin hook to advance the forehead upward and scalp posteriorly, to cause a lift in the brow. Upward counterforce on the forehead is also used. (Reproduced with permission from Chen WP. Oculoplastic surgery: the essentials. New York: Thieme; 2001: 135.)

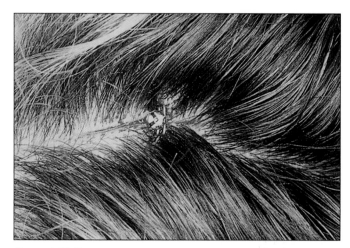

Figure 4.17 Placement of staples behind the screw so that the advanced scalp and forehead position is maintained postoperatively. (Reproduced with permission from Chen WP. Oculoplastic surgery: the essentials. New York: Thieme; 2001: 136.)

Views of a patient before and after endoscopic eyebrow forehead lift are seen in **Figure 4.18**.

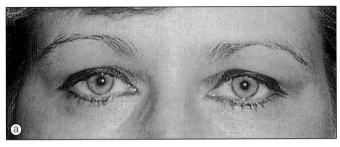 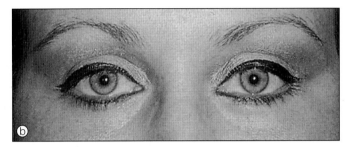

Figure 4.18 Views of a patient before and after endoscopic eyebrow forehead lift. (Reproduced with permission from Chen WP. Oculoplastic surgery: the essentials. New York: Thieme; 2001: 136.)

FURTHER READING

Bostwick J, Eaves FF, Nahai F. Endoscopic plastic surgery. St Louis: Quality Medical Publishing; 1995.

Codner MA. Endoscopic forehead lift. In: McCord CD, ed. Eyelid surgery: principles and techniques. New York: Lippincott-Raven; 1995:368–79.

Daniel RK, Tirkantis B. Endoscopic forehead lift: an operative technique. Plast Reconstr Surg 1996;98:1148–57.

Isse NG. Endoscopic facial rejuvenation: endoforehead, the functional lift, case reports. Aesth Plast Surg 1994;18:21–9.

Kinze DM. An anatomically based study of the mechanism of eyebrow ptosis. Plast Reconstr Surg 1996;97:1321–32.

Kinze DM. Limited incision forehead lift for eyebrow elevation to enhance upper blepharoplasty. Plast Reconstr Surg 1996;97:1334–42.

Lempke BN, Stasior GO. The anatomy of eyebrow ptosis. Arch Ophthalmic 1982;100:981–6.

Loomis MG. Endoscopic brow fixation without brow fixation or miniscrews. Plast Reconstr Surg 1996;98:373–4.

McCord CD. Brow surgery. In: McCord CD, ed. Eyelid surgery: principles and techniques. New York: Lippincott-Raven; 1995:166–70.

Pakkanen M, Salisbury AV, Ersek RA. Biodegradable positive fixation for the endoscopic brow lift. Plast Reconstr Surg 1996;98:1087–90.

Steinsapir KD, Shorr N, Hoenig J, Goldberg RA, Baylis HI, Morrow D. The endoscopic forehead lift. Ophthalmic Plast Reconstr Surg 1998;14:107–18.

Stuzin JM, Wagstrom L, Kawamoto HK, Wolfe SA. Anatomy of the frontal branch of the facial nerve: the significance of the temporal fat pad. Plast Reconstr Surg 1989;83:265–71.

Vasconez LO. Coronal facelift with endoscopic techniques. Plast Surg Forum 1992;15:229.

Upper Blepharoplasty

Chapter 5

William PD Chen

Upper lid blepharoplasty performed without correction of a lax or ptotic eyebrow results in postoperative residual upper lid folds and a narrowing of the spacing between the eyebrow and eyelashes (brow–lash distance). The goal of upper lid blepharoplasty is to remove redundant skinfolds and produce a clear strip of skin above the eyelash line (the eye-shadow space in females).

The following eyebrow procedures are available in conjunction with upper lid blepharoplasty:

- *Internal browpexy* is performed through the upper blepharoplasty incision for correction of laxity in the lateral third of the brow.

- *Endoscopic-assisted eyebrow forehead lift* is used more commonly in females for the nasal two-thirds of the brow and glabellar area

- *Direct eyebrow lift* is used, generally, in males. It involves direct skin incision over the area above the brow (**Fig. 5.1a & b**).

- *Temporal forehead lift* (lateral brow lift) is used for the lateral third of the brow when there is severe skin laxity lateral to the brow, beyond the lateral orbital rim.

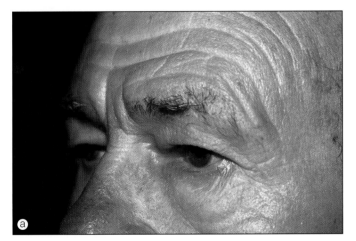

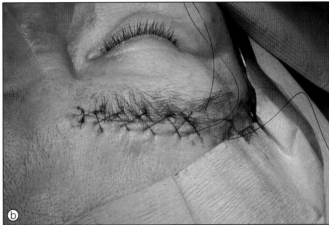

Figure 5.1 (a) Male patient with brow ptosis and voluntary compensation of frontalis muscle.

Figure 5.1 (b) Surgical closure of a direct eyebrow lift.

It is important, when performing upper lid blepharoplasty, for the surgeon to produce an aesthetically pleasing upper eyelid in the patient, but also to use techniques that prevent lagophthalmos of the upper lid, which may cause postoperative exposure symptoms. To achieve this, one may think of the procedure as a three-dimensional reconstruction and reanchoring of the subcutaneous tissues, including orbicularis, orbital septum, preaponeurotic and nasal fat pads, as well as repair of prolapsed lacrimal gland and repair of dehiscence, but with very selective and limited skin excision. **Figure 5.1 c–h** shows examples of variation in upper eyelid crease.

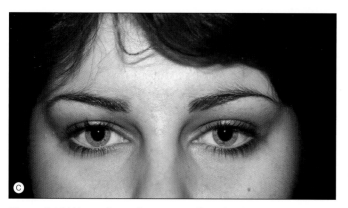

Figure 5.1 (c) Young Caucasian woman with a classical parallel crease in the upper eyelid.

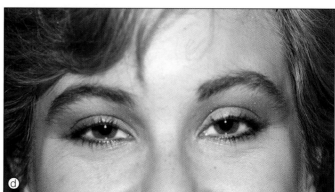

Figure 5.1 (d) Young Caucasian woman with a semilunar crease.

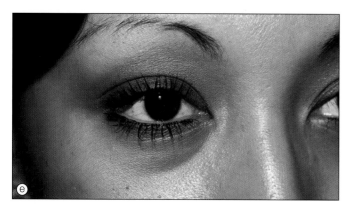

Figure 5.1 (e) Eurasian woman with broad, nasally tapered crease.

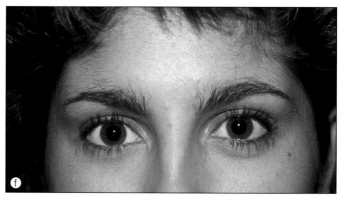

Figure 5.1 (f) Eurasian woman with deep-set eyes and a broad medial extension of her crease.

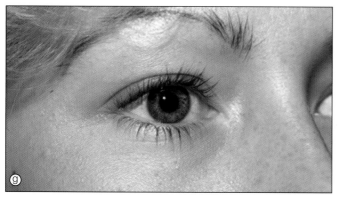

Figure 5.1 (g) Caucasian woman with normal brow-to-crease distance.

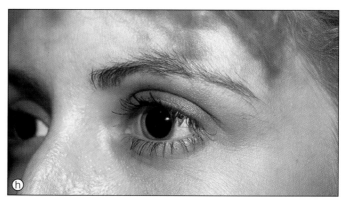

Figure 5.1 (h) Caucasian woman with high crease (or supratarsal sulcus) with low brow position.

Figure 5.2 shows a schematic representation of a cross-sectional view of an upper eyelid with presence of a natural crease.

Generally, females desire a higher lid crease and a more well-defined eye-shadow space and crease than do males. Men, in general, do better with a parallel crease. Adjunctive eyebrow procedures are commonly needed in patients seeking upper lid blepharoplasty. It is possible to produce the goal of crease formation and fold clearance with minimal skin excision when adequate brow stabilization and debulking of the upper lid are performed.

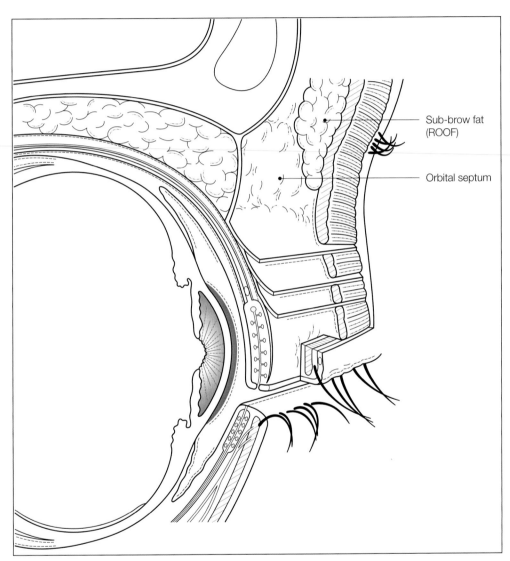

Sub-brow fat (ROOF)

Orbital septum

Figure 5.2 Cross-sectional view of an upper lid with crease presence. (Reproduced with permission from Chen WP. Oculoplastic surgery: the essentials. New York: Thieme; 2001: 212.)

Surgical Technique

At the mid portion of the upper lid crease, the upper lid is anesthetized through skin-subcutaneously with no more than 2mL of 2% Xylocaine with 1:100 000 dilution epinephrine, through a 30-gauge needle. The anesthetic solution is lightly massaged several times to spread it evenly across medially and laterally. After 2 minutes to allow for vasoconstriction to set in, the surgical field is draped. A corneal protector is applied. I prefer to inject the nasal fat pad quadrant only after I have reached the preaponeurotic space, with an open view.

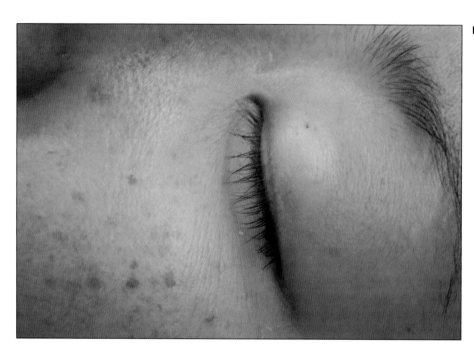

Figure 5.3

 Clinical pearls

- Avoid using large-gauge needles during injection.

- Avoid any repeated passage through the orbicularis layers to reduce the chance of bleeding.

- Inject slowly, from a perpendicular orientation over the central preseptal area of the orbicularis; then massage to both sides.

- Use diluted Xylocaine mix (see Chapter 3), or use bicarbonate supplement to decrease stinging sensation from the acidity of the full-strength injection.

 Pitfalls

- Regional nerve block is often unnecessary, as some patients are bordered by transient torsional diplopia and ptosis from involvement of the levator muscle and superior oblique tendon.

Designing the skin excision

The central position of the upper lid crease is marked centrally at 8.5 to 10mm above the lashes in females, in a semicircular configuration. Medially, it tapers down to 5mm from the lashes and may angle upward in the vicinity of the upper punctum. Laterally, the crease line is carried to about 6mm from the lash line and then the marking is angled upward, pointing toward the end of the brow.

In men, I prefer to mark the crease centrally at 8–9mm, and in a parallel shape. The medial extent of the line of incision is about 7mm and the lateral extent about 8mm from the lash line, rendering it more of a parallel crease shape.

For Asians, the upper crease is measured. The central height of the tarsus is similarly measured by everting the tarsus. If the two measurements are identical, the patient's original crease line is used as the lower marking for incision. If the current crease measures more than the central tarsal height, this author prefers to transcribe the tarsal height measurement onto the skin side as a yardstick to the proper height for the new crease.

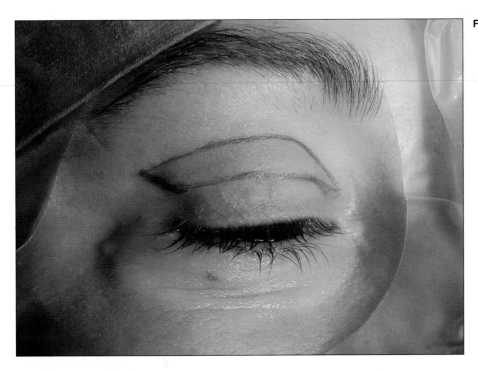

Figure 5.4

 Clinical pearls

- Allow adequate amount of time for anesthetic solution to spread out and egress; this will reduce the tissue distortion.

- If the tissues are marked before injection, one tends to make an excessively high incision and often inadvertently injure the levator. This can cause cicatricial lagophthalmos on downgaze as well as upgaze.

- The use of hyaluronidase (Wydase), when available, is a helpful adjunct towards achieving the correct incision height and ultimately the crease height.

 Pitfalls

- In men, the crease looks best if it is close to and along the superior tarsal border.

- Avoid excessive fat removal, especially in men, as it will exaggerate the sulcus.

For marking the upper line of the skin excision ellipse, the bunching technique is used only at the lateral canthus. The proper amount of bunching in this area should show some slight eversion of lashes. One may maximize the skin excision laterally and should minimize the skin excision centrally and nasally. Any lagophthalmos in the upper lid is poorly tolerated if it occurs in the central or nasal portion of the lid. One way of ensuring symmetry in the final upper lid crease position is to measure the distance of the superior line of incision from the brow hairs above.

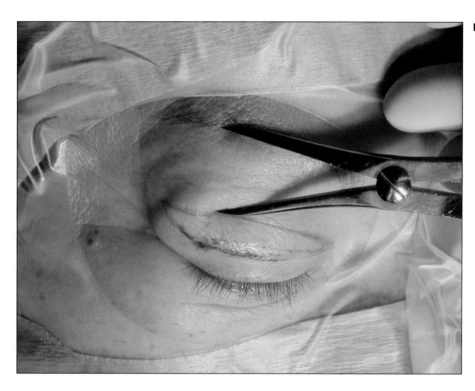

Figure 5.5

 Clinical pearls

- The superior line of the ellipse should be measured from the inferior edge of the brow hairs and generally is located at the juncture of the thick and thin skin of the upper lid (**Fig. 5.5**). Equal distances from the upper line of incision to the brow hairs will give even creases postoperatively if the brow positions are symmetrical on both sides.

- To create symmetry in an asymmetric condition, an asymmetric amount of excision has to be performed on the two sides. One should match and equalize the pretarsal distances (crease-to-lashes) as well as the brow-to-crease distances bilaterally.

 Pitfalls

- Bunching to determine the amount of skin removal should not be used in the central or nasal portion of the eyelid because the amount of skin excision in these areas should be conservative. If bunching is used medially and centrally, one risks excising too much tissue, which may result in anterior lamella shortage.

- Avoid high incision and fixation as it may impinge on the levator muscle's ability to contract (upgaze) and relax (downgaze).

- Avoid excessive excision of skin medially, as it will result in cicatricial ectropion.

Skin incision

Debulking involves removal of the marked area of skin, muscle, and septum, and removal of eyelid fat. After the skin incision has been marked, pressure on the globe allows the eyelid skin to be on stretch and skin-subcutaneous incisions are carried out with a No. 15 blade over the superior as well as the lower line of incisions. Light application of wetfield cautery is used to control any bleeding from small vessels along the skin incisions. I prefer to use a Bovie cautery with a fine needle tip to traverse through the orbicularis and septum along the superior incision, in a slightly beveled fashion.

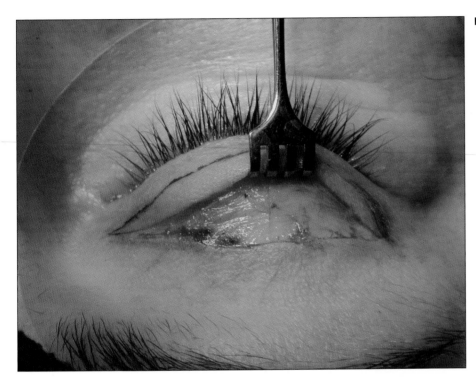

Figure 5.6

 Clinical pearls

- The skin incision using a No. 15 blade is only skin deep, through full-thickness dermis.

- There is a tendency to make the incision on the skin based on the outer border of the marked incision lines. To counteract this tendency, concentrate on following the incision based on the outer edge of the lower line of incision (the crease incision), and to go on the inner border of the upper marked line. This gives a safer margin of error – the crease-to-lash distance (pretarsal platform) will not be over-exaggerated into a very high upper lid crease, nor will the crease-to-brow distance be overly shortened. The total amount of resected skin–muscle–septum will remain the same as what was intended and marked.

 Pitfalls

- Carefully use the radiofrequency unit in making the skin incision as one may go through deeper muscular layers inadvertently.

Transection through the upper incision line's orbicularis layer

A Bovie cutting needle is used to transect through the orbicularis layer to reach the orbital septum. Typically, a rent is created through the septum and protruding preaponeurotic fat pad can be observed. Bipolar cautery is used to cauterize bleeding small vessels in the muscle layers.

Blunt-tipped Westcott spring scissors are used to open the septum medially and laterally in a transverse fashion.

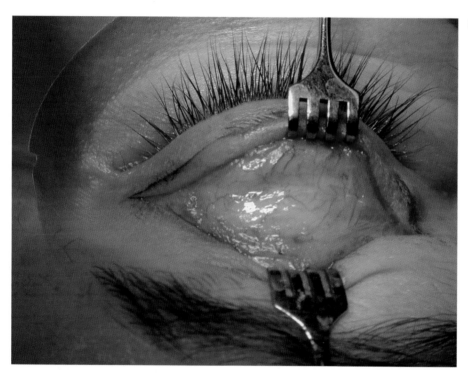

Figure 5.7

 Clinical pearls

■ The beveling upward of the direction of cutting (using the Bovie tip) through the orbicularis layer along the upper line of incision allows a more uniform distribution of the Bovie's thermal stress as well as directing it away from the overlying skin incision.

■ This allows access to the preaponeurotic space at a higher level from the superior tarsal border, thereby making it more likely to reach and open the orbital septum safely and without injury to the underlying levator aponeurosis.

 Pitfalls

■ Be extra cautious in controlling small vessel bleeding from cut edges of the orbicularis. Untreated vessels often result in unsightly hematomas postoperatively.

The skin–orbicularis flap is retracted inferiorly using a Blair retractor, exposing the preaponeurotic fat, junctional fat (transitional fat), and, occasionally, the nasal fat pad. I use forceps and scissors to clear the preaponeurotic fat from the underlying levator aponeurosis. A small infiltrate of Xylocaine may be injected to the back of the preaponeurotic fat pad at this time, as well as over the nasal fat pad region.

Depending on the amount of excessive and prolapsing preaponeurotic fat, part of it or most of it may be excised. A combination of bipolar and monopolar Bovie cautery, as well as Westcott scissors are used to transect the fat pedicle a small portion at a time, until the whole amount is removed, in a careful and controlled fashion.

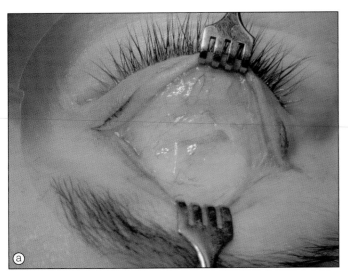

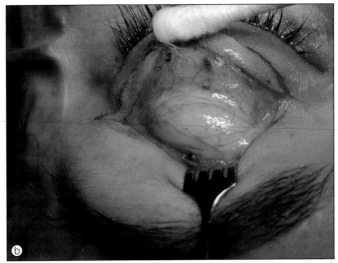

Figure 5.8

Clinical pearls

■ Using a hemostat to apply the clamp–cut–cautery technique of fat excision often yields some level of discomfort or a reactive jerk from the patient.

■ After 0.5mL of Xylocaine has been applied, the gentle teasing and cutting using the combination of bipolar as well as Bovie cautery is usually very atraumatic. It allows an even distribution of fat excision across the width of the preaponeurotic space.

■ It is important to reposit the remaining fat pedicle carefully into the antero-superior orbital space, under the orbital septum. I try to avoid directly placing the cut edge of the fat near any cut edges of the orbicularis or orbital septum to avoid any possibility of cicatrix formation.

■ In the prominent-eyed patient, one should be conservative in preaponeurotic fat removal so as not to accentuate the height of the upper crease, which may make the eye appear even more prominent.

Pitfalls

■ Avoid deep placement of the Bovie needle into the supero-medial orbital space behind the orbital rim, to avoid injury to the trochlea and the superior oblique tendon.

■ The clamp–cut–cautery maneuver of fat excision may tend to focus the fat removal over only the central one-third or one-half of the preaponeurotic space. It may create a central 'divot' of excision.

Located over the medial extent of the incision is a distinctive and separate fat pad – the nasal fat pad. When clinically prominent, it may be excised. A Blair retractor is placed in the inner canthus, and with pressure on the globe, an incision is made with a cutting Bovie needle through the capsule covering the pale-yellow nasal fat. The nasal fat pad is teased out with the forceps and the cotton applicator stick. Often a prominent vessel is seen and it can be selectively cauterized with bipolar cautery; then, a combination of scissors and coagulation Bovie is used to excise the nasal fat pad. Bipolar cautery is used to reduce the fat and to cauterize the vessels. The fat is reinspected for any potential bleeding vessels.

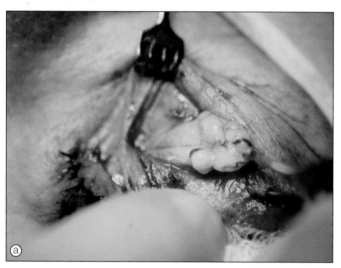

Figure 5.9 (a) Nasal fat pad.

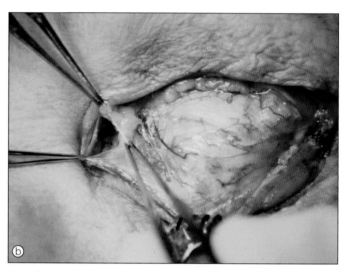

Figure 5.9 (b) Space after nasal fat pad has been excised.

Clinical pearls

■ It is important to recognize and identify the much larger vessels here in the nasal fat pad, so that it is adequately cauterized before allowing it to retract into the deep orbital space.

■ The placement and successive replacement of a retractor, as well as gentle ballotment on the globe, helps in identifying the nasal fat pad.

■ An application of bipolar cautery (instead of Bovie cautery) on the fat pad's capsule prior to incision with Westcott scissors is an alternative to what was stated above. It helps to open the nasal fat pocket without having to use Bovie cautery in this important sector of the orbital space, where the superior oblique trochlea and tendon are located.

Pitfalls

■ Deep placement of the Bovie cautery tip in the nasal fat pad space is to be avoided. There is the potential for pain and discomfort, as well as injury to the fourth-nerve structures.

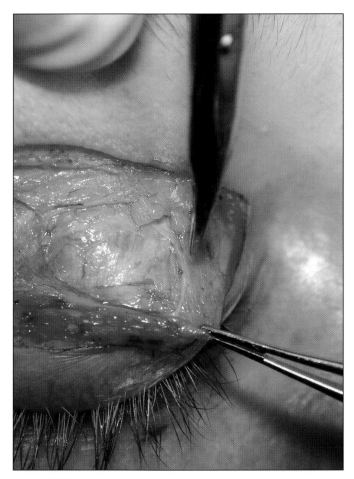

Figure 5.10

There is a separate area of fat in the transitional zone between the preaponeurotic fat and the white nasal fat. This transitional fat (junctional fat) invests the conjoined septum and extension of Whitnall's ligament that forms the interpad septum.

 Clinical pearls

■ Removal of the transitional fat will produce a depression in the eyelid crease nasally; thus, it should not be removed.

 Pitfalls

■ Avoid inadvertent weakening of the medial aspect of the levator aponeurosis. Dehiscence may lead to segmental ptosis.

An open view of the preaponeurotic platform is now possible. If there should be any prolapsed lobe of the lacrimal gland (**Fig. 5.11a**), it can be repositioned by first securing its capsule with a 5-0 Vicryl, then passing the needle to a point behind the supero-nasal orbital rim, taking a bite of the inner periorbita within the lacrimal gland fossa. When tied, the suture should retract the lacrimal gland behind the orbital rim (**Fig. 5.11b**).

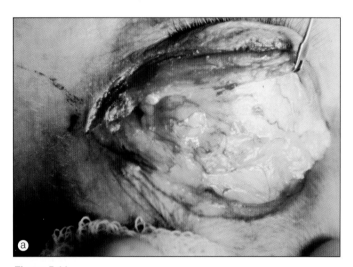
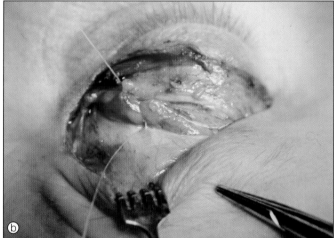

Figure 5.11

<table>
<tr><td>

○ Clinical pearls

■ If left without repositioning, the prolapsed lacrimal gland tends to leave a bulge that is noticeable and unsightly over the lateral preseptal area of the eyelid.

■ Never excise any portion of the lacrimal gland lobe.

■ Do not cauterize it in an attempt to reduce the lacrimal gland.

</td><td>

! Pitfalls

■ The repositioning stitch should engage only the capsule of the gland as you reposition it behind the orbital rim in the lacrimal gland fossa.

■ Do not encircle the lacrimal gland lobe with any suture element.

</td></tr>
</table>

After fat reduction, the myocutaneous flap (redundant upper lid hooding) that is now hinged along the superior tarsal border can be trimmed along such through the lower line of the incision. (The more traditional blepharoplasty stages involve removal of the skin and orbicularis muscle in two steps, as well as the opening of the septum as a third step.) The flap is elevated with gentle traction, separating the edges of the skin incision while it is being excised. I use a Bovie tip on cutting mode to tease (cut) through the orbicularis that is holding the myocutaneous flap down along the superior tarsal border. Straight scissors may also be used, slanting away from the insertions of the levator aponeurosis so as not to disrupt them. Crease sutures that will be used in closure will repair any dehiscences in the levator, but it is wise to avoid any disruption in the levator attachments. Potential bleeding areas are in the orbicularis and subcutaneous layer of the lower crease incision. The pretarsal skin is retracted with cotton applicator sticks to expose the inferior edge of the pretarsal orbicularis muscle, and bipolar cautery is used to cauterize any bleeding vessels in this area.

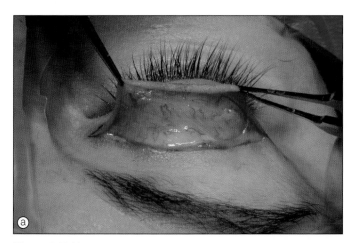

Figure 5.12 (a)

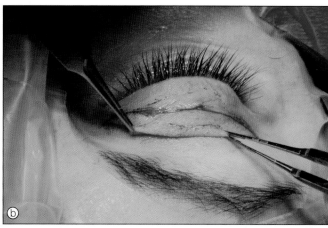

Figure 5.12 (b)

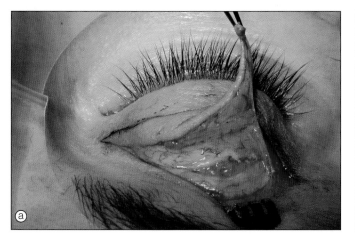

Figure 5.12 (c)

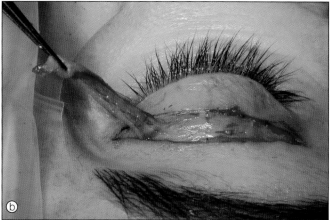

Figure 5.12 (d)

◑ Clinical pearls

■ It is important to be conservative during the first passage using the cutting Bovie tip as you sever the flap of redundant skin–orbicularis tissues along the lower skin incision. This will allow you some separation from the underlying levator.

■ One may elect to further clean up the strip of orbicularis/fascial tissues that appear excessive and overlie the superior tarsal border, by further excision along the lower skin edge.

■ It is helpful to pause and control bleeders from the orbicularis with bipolar cautery as you cut along with the Bovie cautery.

■ At the lateral end of the myocutaneous flap, I try to shallow my plane of excision to reduce my chance of cutting across any of the larger arterioles present within the periorbital orbicularis muscle.

! Pitfalls

■ Do not apply any coagulative Bovie cautery as it may excessively char and damage the levator muscle fibers.

■ If one encounters partial dehiscence of the levator, it should be repaired with 7-0 silk or 6-0 Vicryl.

Before final skin closure, the interpad septum is lysed to reduce tethering of closure of the upper lid (**Fig. 5.13**).

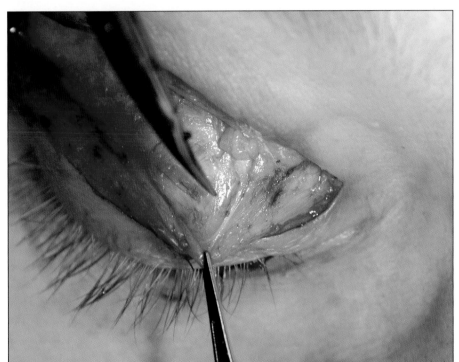

Figure 5.13 Lysis of interpad septum.

Crease fixation

For patients who desire to have further enhancement of the upper lid crease, the crease may be reinforced by applying five to six 6-0 silk stitches, placing them in an interrupted fashion from the lower skin incision, including a small bite of the levator aponeurosis directly above the superior tarsal border, to upper lid skin edge.

Instead of skin–levator–skin interrupted stitches, an approach using additional 6-0 Vicryl sutures may be used to fixate the pretarsal skin–muscle edge to the levator aponeurosis. It is applied just 1 mm below the inferior skin edge, in a transcutaneous fashion and picking up a bite of the aponeurosis above the superior tarsal border. The knot is then double-tied over the anterior pretarsal skin surface. It is usually applied in three locations: central, medial, and lateral third of the wound. It corrects any dehiscence of the levator that could have occurred with excision of the myocutaneous-septal flap. The three knots are cut away at 1 week after the operation, while each of their residual loops are left behind underneath the pretarsal tissues to promote some wound reaction.

This maneuver:

- ensures crease position; and

- prevents ptosis that may occur from undetected injury to the levator.

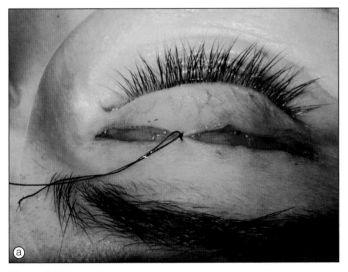 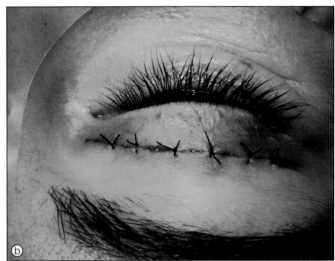

Figure 5.14

 Clinical pearls

- Without crease fixation and anchoring, the upper lid preseptal skin muscle layers may balloon down and cover over the pretarsal platform space.

Skin closure

The upper blepharoplasty wound is normally closed with either 6-0 nylon, 6-0 Prolene, or 7-0 silk (**Fig. 5.15a & b**). I favor starting at the medial end of the incision and working towards the lateral end, as the wound stress is greater at the lateral end.

At the lateral end of the upper blepharoplasty incision, I use an interlocking 'baseball stitch' (first popularized by Dr Clinton McCord) to terminate the closure. Essentially, it is a far–far–near–near stitch that is then interlocked to give stability and symmetry to the wound edges. (Similarly, I use this stitching in the lateral portion of lower blepharoplasty closure.)

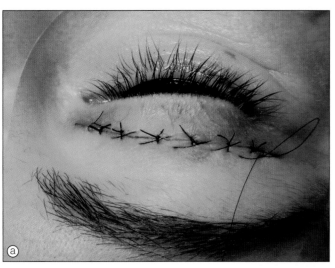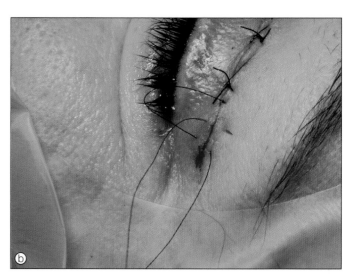

Figure 5.15

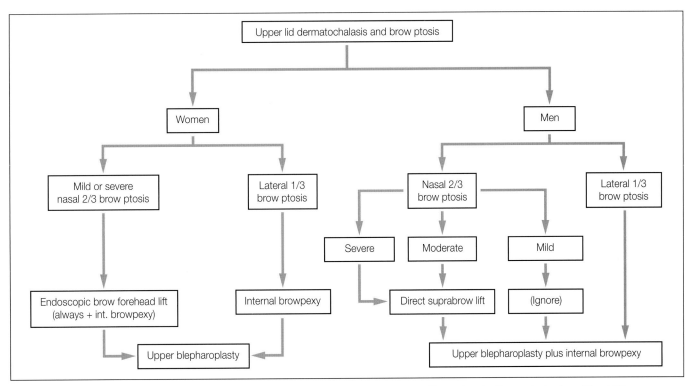

Figure 5.16 Decision tree for management of upper lid dermatochalasis and eyebrow ptosis. (Reproduced with permission from Chen WP. Oculoplastic surgery: the essentials. New York: Thieme; 2001: 145.)

The flowchart in **Figure 5.16** outlines the approach to the treatment of patients with upper eyelid dermatochalasis and brow ptosis.

FURTHER READING

McCord CD. Techniques in blepharoplasty. Ophthalmic Surg 1979;10:40–55.

McCord CD. Upper blepharoplasty. In: McCord CD, ed. Eyelid surgery: principles and techniques. New York: Lippincott-Raven; 1995;179–95.

Sheen JH. Supratarsal fixation in upper blepharoplasty. Plast Reconstr Surg 1974;54:424–31.

Direct Browlift, Internal Browpexy, Browplasty

Chapter 6

William PD Chen

In the evaluation of patients with upper eyelid skin redundancy and hooding, it is important to note the upper brow position and check for eyebrow ptosis. The upper eyebrow normally rests above the superior orbital rim in females and at the level of the supra-orbital rim in males. With aging, the brow may sag down to below the orbital rim. A ptotic brow can gravitate into the upper lid skin area, creating a secondary eyelid hooding, which is relieved when the eyebrow is repositioned to its normal location. Symptoms may include visual fatigue, visual field obstruction, and fatigue of the forehead muscles, as well as headaches. This process of brow ptosis also produces a narrowed spacing between the eyebrow hairs and the lashes, which can cause a frowning appearance in the patient. The presence of brow ptosis therefore needs to be addressed either before the blepharoplasty or handled concurrently. Because of this sequence, the eyebrow procedures are described first in this atlas.

The following eyebrow procedures that are commonly used in conjunction with upper lid blepharoplasty are covered in detail in this chapter:

- *Internal browpexy* is performed through the upper blepharoplasty incision for correction of laxity in the lateral third of the brow. It is commonly used by itself in conjunction with upper lid blepharoplasty or used as a supplement to the endoscopic eyebrow forehead lift or the direct eyebrow lift for elevation of the lateral third or tail of the brow.

- *Endoscopic-assisted eyebrow forehead lift* (see Chapter 4) is used more commonly in females for the nasal two-thirds of the brow and glabellar area. (It is commonly supplemented with the internal browpexy.)

- *Direct eyebrow lift* is used, generally, in males. It involves direct skin incision over the area above the brow. It is also commonly supplemented with the internal browpexy, which corrects for lateral brow ptosis.

- *Temporal forehead lift* is used for the lateral third of the brow when there is severe skin laxity lateral to the brow, beyond the lateral orbital rim. Performed through a subgaleal approach, it is commonly used as a supplement to the cheeklift procedure.

A sagging eyebrow can be corrected by a *direct brow lift*. After the eyebrow area is locally anesthetized, an above-brow incision line is designed from the medial to the lateral extent of the upper eyebrow hair, in a gentle curve with a slight lateral flare upward. A segment of the ptotic forehead skin, usually between 8 and 10mm, is marked out parallel to this lower incision. A No. 15 blade is used to incise the upper and lower brow markings. The strip of ptotic forehead skin and subcutaneous tissue, down to the level of the frontalis muscle, is excised using cutting Bovie cautery with a needle tip. The deep frontalis muscles are reapproximated to those at the deep plane of the upper incisional edge, using multiple interrupted 4-0 Polydek sutures (ME-2 needle, Deknatel). The subcutaneous tissues are then closed using subcuticular placement of 5-0 Vicryl. The skin is closed with 6-0 nylon in an interlocking running stitch. The nylon stitches may be kept in place for 10–14 days.

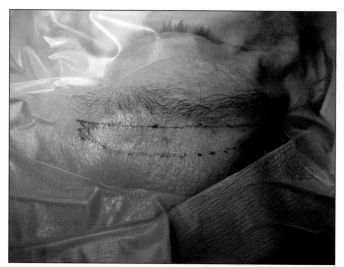

Figure 6.1

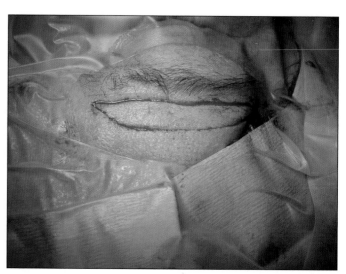

Figure 6.2

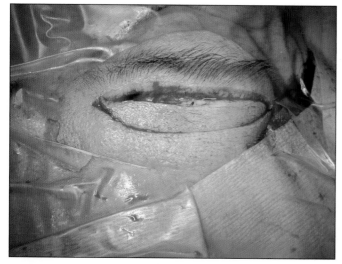

Figure 6.3

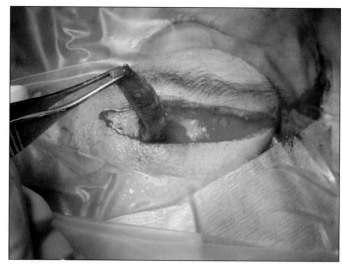

Figure 6.4

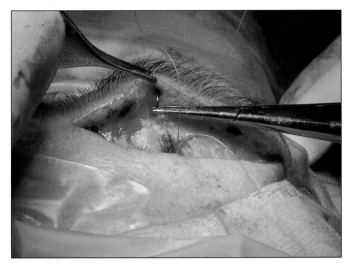

Figure 6.5

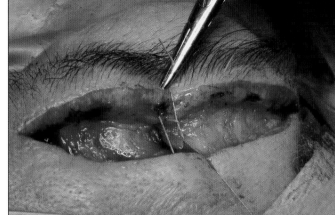

Figure 6.6

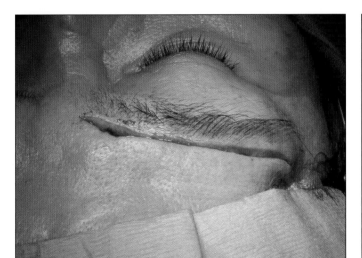

Figure 6.7

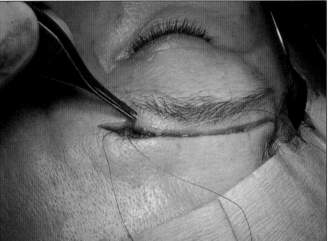

Figure 6.8

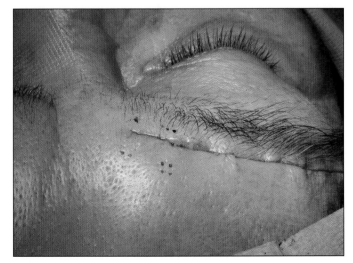

Figure 6.9

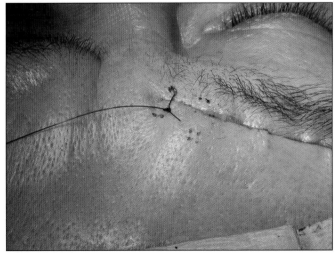

Figure 6.10

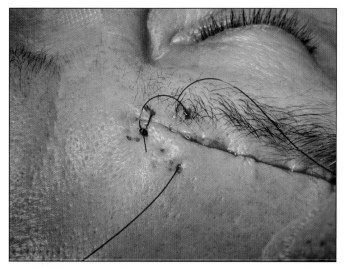

Figure 6.11

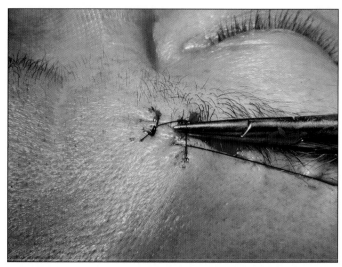

Figure 6.12

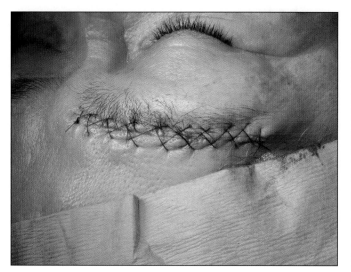

Figure 6.13

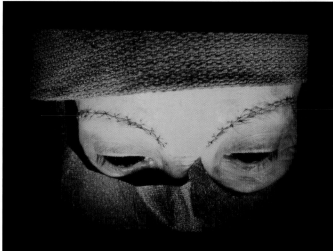

Figure 6.14

 Clinical pearls

- Direct browlift is well suited for men with a receding hairline, as it avoids further migration of the hairline.

- The wound can be easily disguised in patients with deep forehead furrows.

- The medial incision lines should taper well before the medial border of the brow hair is reached.

- The sutures need to be left in longer to avoid wound spreading due to the strength of frontalis muscle.

- Wound edges need to be closed in a slightly everted and tension-free fashion.

! Pitfalls

- A prominent incision line will form medially in the thick skin of the forehead if the incision is extended too far medially.

- One should avoid anchoring any of the deeper plane tissues to the underlying periosteum as this will cause an immobile brow.

- Often, patients may complain of hypoesthesia over the forehead region.

A lateral brow sag can be corrected by a *direct lateral brow lift*, with the excision of the ptotic forehead skin concentrating on the lateral extent of the supra-brow region (**Fig. 6.15**). Closure may be performed using baseball stitching or interrupted sutures.

Figure 6.15

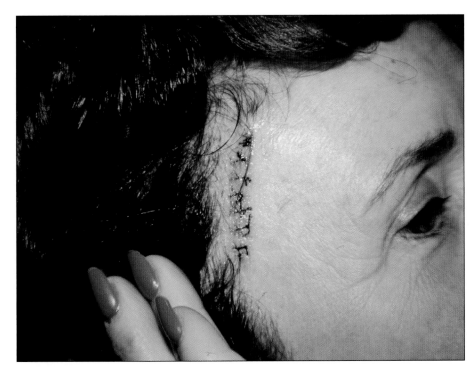

Clinical pearls

■ A direct lateral brow lift is great for lateral sagging of the tail of the eyebrows.

■ The incision is well hidden behind the hairline.

The *mid-forehead brow lift* is another variation of the direct brow lift. It is suitable for individuals with deep furrows of the forehead and significant brow ptosis, and in patients who would benefit from forward advancement of the hairline. The procedure is especially appropriate for men with receding hairline or baldness (**Fig. 6.16**).

After the forehead is anesthetized with frontal nerve block and local infiltration, McCord mentions that when planning for the skin incisions, one should try to find two furrows and plan to make the initial incision in the upper one and develop the flap for advancement inferiorly. If the amount of forehead skin to be resected coincides with a lower furrow, this will result in an ideal scar (**Fig. 6.17**).

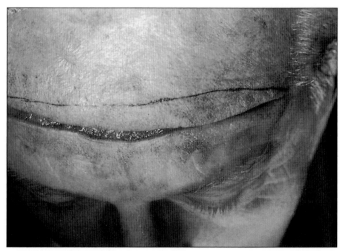

Figure 6.17 Coronal forehead lift, midforehead incision. Surgical view showing the area of skin and forehead tissue to be excised in this patient. (Reproduced with permission from McCord CD. Eyelid surgery: principles and techniques. Philadelphia: Lippincott-Raven; 1995: 177.)

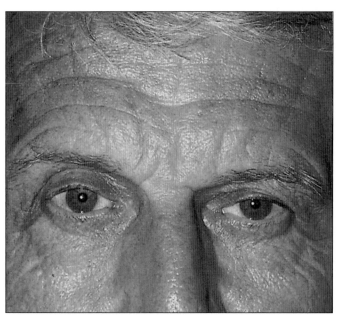

Figure 6.16 Coronal forehead lift, midforehead incision. Patient preoperatively. (Reproduced with permission from McCord CD. Eyelid surgery: principles and techniques. Philadelphia: Lippincott-Raven; 1995: 177.)

The resection of skin and development of the flap can occur in either the subgaleal or subcutaneous plane. The *subgaleal* flap is easier to elevate and to close with less scar. However, it transects the sensory nerves, with significant forehead numbness postoperatively. The *subcutaneous* flap does not cause quite as much sensory loss but closure is more difficult, with tension on the skin edges. When the wound is closed, separate galeal closure is needed if it is incised. The forehead skin is closed with everting vertical mattress sutures (4-0 Prolene) and vertical mattress sutures (6-0 nylon) (**Fig. 6.18a & b**).

Typically, the second forehead wrinkle tends to cross the midline; therefore, the tissues between the second and the third forehead wrinkles are excised, counting from the brow upward.

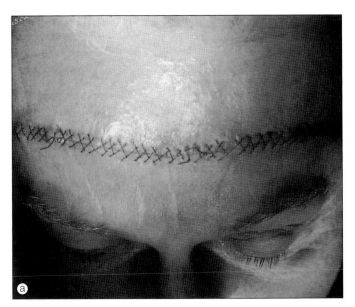
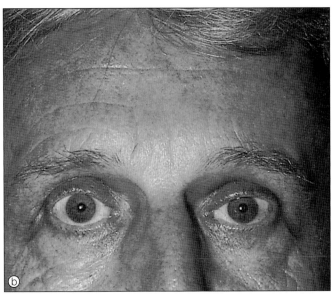

Figure 6.18 Coronal forehead lift, midforehead incision. (a) The skin segment has been excised in this patient with closure of the galea and vertical mattress skin closure. (b) Same patient, 6 weeks postoperatively. (Reproduced with permission from McCord CD. Eyelid surgery: principles and techniques. Philadelphia: Lippincott-Raven; 1995: 177.)

Optional Lateral Brow Procedures Performed in Conjunction with Upper Blepharoplasty Approach

If there are certain aging changes in the brow that will not be corrected by upper lid blepharoplasty alone, and lateral brow procedures are appropriate, the following can be used at this stage of the upper lid blepharoplasty.

Internal browpexy

If there is enough laxity in the temporal one-third of the brow so that there is concern that residual skinfolds may persist there or that the lateral eye-shadow space may not form well postoperatively, an internal browpexy should be performed laterally. This is an effective, convenient procedure for correction of mild-to-moderate brow ptosis that can be performed through the wound of, and at the same time as, an upper blepharoplasty.

Steps of browpexy

Three to four double 4-0 Prolene sutures are used. Each of the sutures is passed transcutaneously from the skin below the ptotic brow through the eyelid skin and exiting into the sub-brow space over the superior orbital rim (**Fig. 6.19a**). The exit site under the brow flap is marked with methylene blue. The needle is then passed through the periosteum at a location 5–10mm above the superior orbital rim (**Fig. 6.19b**). The suture is then passed to the underside of the brow flap, near the methylene blue marking. The transcutaneous end of the suture is then passed through and exits under the brow flap. When the two ends are tied, this will result in the lower boundary of the ptotic brow being elevated back to a point above the superior orbital rim, correcting the brow ptosis (**Fig. 6.20**).

The upper blepharoplasty wound may then be closed as described in the previous chapter.

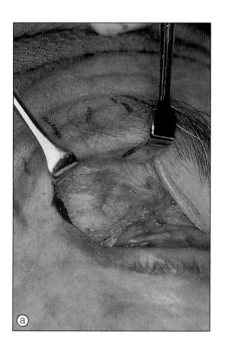
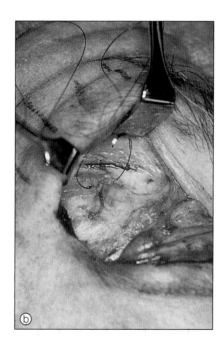

Figure 6.19 Internal browpexy of right brow. (a) Dissection in the planes superficial to the periosteum and deep temporal fascia, exposing the juncture of the deep temporal fascia to the skull, the fusion point, and the orbital ligament. (b) A fixating 4-0 Prolene suture has been placed in the deep temporal fascia at its point of fusion to the skull periosteum. The suture will subsequently be inserted into the fat and orbicularis fibers under the flap at the level of the inferior eyebrow hairs and then tied for brow support. (Reproduced with permission from Chen WP. Oculoplastic surgery: the essentials. New York: Thieme; 2001: 129–30.)

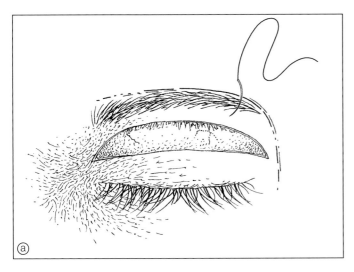

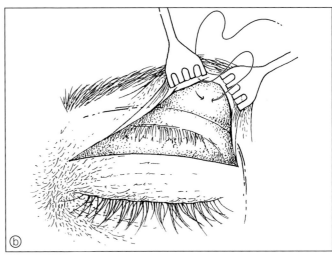

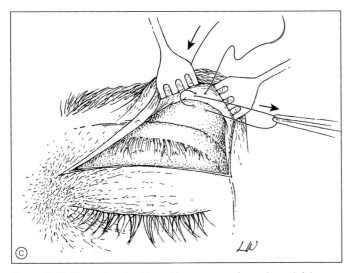

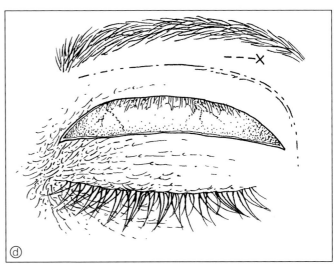

Figure 6.20 Steps showing internal browpexy performed over left brow.

Browplasty

Excessive lateral brow fullness or prominence can sometimes be a major complaint of the patient presenting for an upper lid blepharoplasty. This excessive fullness may not corrected by the usual excision of skin and muscle using the standard upper lid blepharoplasty technique. This fullness can be caused by a prominent bony superior rim, but is most commonly caused by superabundance of the retro-orbicularis oculi brow fat (ROOF). When the ROOF layer hypertrophies, it may extend downward into the eyelid proper, where it becomes preseptal fat. In these patients, sculpting and surgical excision of the ROOF can allow reduction in this overly prominent area. It is performed in conjunction with upper blepharoplasty through the same lid crease access.

Approach

It is performed by approaching the fat pads in a sub-orbicularis plane towards the superior orbital rim and as far lateral as the lateral orbital rim. An internal browpexy may be performed at the same time, if necessary, to correct for any brow ptosis.

Surgical technique

The upper edge of the blepharoplasty incision is retracted to expose the brow fat at the superior orbital rim (**Fig. 6.21**). Two Blair rake retractors are inserted to retract the skin–muscle edge. The area of fat on the rim to be removed is marked with methylene blue and is then excised by grasping the fat with Adson forceps and dissecting it free of the periosteum using the Bovie coagulating needle. Dissection should not extend nasally to the superior orbital notch so as to avoid damaging the nerves and vessels in that area. The dissection is performed until one is approximately 1cm above the rim. A segment of fat usually measuring 1.0–1.5cm in vertical dimension and then tapering nasally and temporally is removed (**Fig. 6.22**). The resection should extend laterally to the frontozygomatic suture. The periosteum is left intact to prevent the occurrence of postoperative adhesions that may hinder brow movement. Additional redundant skin may be produced after brow fat excision, and any redundant fold should be excised to prevent double folding in the crease area.

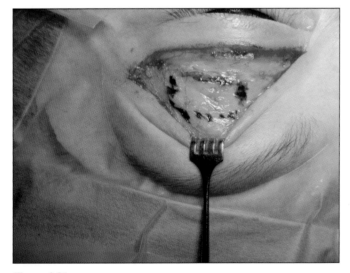

Figure 6.21

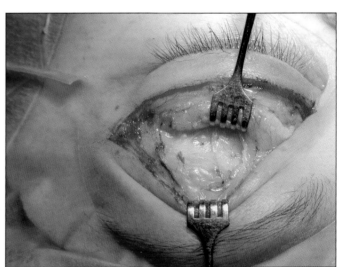

Figure 6.22

FURTHER READING

Bostwick J, Eaves FF, Nahai F. Endoscopic plastic surgery. St Louis: Quality Medical Publishing; 1995.

Codner MA. Endoscopic forehead lift. In: McCord CD, ed. Eyelid surgery: principles and techniques. New York: Lippincott-Raven; 1995:368–79.

Daniel RK, Tirkantits B. Endoscopic forehead lift: an operative technique. Plast Reconstr Surg 1996;98:1148–57.

Isse NG. Endoscopic facial rejuvenation: endoforehead, the functional lift, case reports. Aesth Plast Surg 1994;18:21–9.

Kinze DM. An anatomically based study of the mechanism of eyebrow ptosis. Plast Reconstr Surg 1996;97:1321–32.

Kinze DM. Limited incision forehead lift for eyebrow elevation to enhance upper blepharoplasty. Plast Reconstr Surg 1996;97:1334–42.

Lempke BN, Stasior GO. The anatomy of eyebrow ptosis. Arch Ophthalmic 1982;100:981–6.

Loomis MG. Endoscopic brow fixation without brow fixation or miniscrews. Plast Reconstr Surg 1996;98:373–4.

McCord CD, Doxanas MT. Browplasty and browpexy: an adjunct to blepharoplasty. Plast Reconstr Surg 1990;86:248–54.

McCord CD. Brow surgery. In: McCord CD, ed. Eyelid surgery: principles and techniques. New York: Lippincott-Raven; 1995:166–170.

Pakkanen M, Salisbury AV, Ersek RA. Biodegradable positive fixation for the endoscopic brow lift. Plast Reconstr Surg 1996;98:1087–90.

Steinsapir KD, Shorr N, Hoenig J, Goldberg RA, Baylis HI, Morrow D. The endoscopic forehead lift. Ophthalmic Plast Reconstr Surg 1998;14:107–18.

Stuzin JM, Wagstrom L, Kawamoto HK, Wolfe SA. Anatomy of the frontal branch of the facial nerve: the significance of the temporal fat pad. Plast Reconstr Surg 1989;83:265–71.

Vasconez LO. Coronal facelift with endoscopic techniques. Plast Surg Forum 1992;15:229.

Asian Blepharoplasty of the Upper Eyelid

Chapter 7

William PD Chen

The main reasons why Asians without an upper eyelid crease may elect to have a crease placed have been discussed in Chapter 1. There are many fallacies in discussions of eyelid surgery for Asians. The conventional view that Asian eyelid surgery started only after the Second World War, with industrialization and westernization of Asia, is in my opinion erroneous. There has always been a demand for this type of cosmetic surgery in Asia, the first 20 descriptions of the double eyelid crease procedure being reported in the Japanese medical literature between 1896 and 1940. In the Western Hemisphere over the last 40 years, there has been a simultaneous rise in demand as more Asians leave their homeland and settle abroad. Demography shows that Asians seeking eyelid crease procedures are a relatively young, affluent, and educated group. However, despite being educated, the patients' understanding of what they want, and of what can be achieved, may not be equivalent to the surgeon's own beliefs. They may not be aware of the normal wound healing processes and have unrealistic expectations. In addition, the physician may not be fully informed of the nuances of this specialized and peculiar aspect of aesthetic eyelid surgery. Most of the complications and suboptimal results may be linked to a lack of communication between the patient and the surgeon, and the failure of the surgeon to observe certain basic concepts and hidden dangers.

One of the most common fallacies is the notion that most Asians do not have an upper eyelid crease. This may be because, typically, only those subjects without a crease would consult an aesthetic surgeon. The lid crease occurs in varying incidence among different ethnic subsets of Asians,[1] whether Chinese, Korean, or Japanese, etc. It shows provincial and geographic variance (e.g. northern versus southern Chinese; Japanese who are from the northern island of Hokkaido versus those from the more southern province of Kyushu). Overall, among Han ethnic

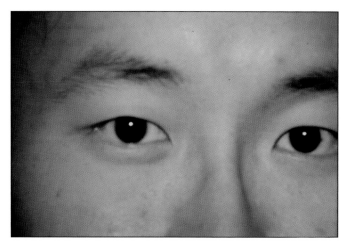

Figure 7.1 Single eyelid without upper lid crease.

groups (Chinese, Koreans, and Japanese), the prevalence of a crease is 50% (**Fig. 7.1**). Consequently, one in two Asians is likely to have an upper eyelid crease. This ratio holds true even among parents and their offspring – for instance, two out of four siblings will have an upper eyelid crease, or one of the two parents will have a crease. The crease occurs in approximate correlation to the height (vertical dimension) of the superior tarsal plate, as measured over the central portion above the pupillary aperture. Asians are, in general, smaller in physical dimensions relative to non-Asians. Their tarsal plate height averages 6.5–8.0mm, and the upper lid crease, if present, is usually not greater than this distance from the eyelid margin (ciliary border). With respect to the depth of inward folding of the crease line, the crease is not any less prominent in Asians as compared with non-Asians. One of the reasons that the lateral canthus appears more upslanted may be the presence medially of a fold of skin over the crease, partially blocking the upper medial half of the palpebral fissure. There have been recent reports describing a higher lateral canthal position among certain ethnic subset of Asians, although one certainly cannot deduce or generalize this finding to all Asians.

The current hypothesis regarding the lid crease is that it results from the presence of subcutaneous terminal interdigitations of the levator aponeurosis in the pretarsal as well as along the superior tarsal border area. The distal terminations of the levator aponeurosis fibers blend into the intermuscular septal and connective tissue fibers of the pretarsal orbicularis oculi muscle,[2] resulting in an infolding when the levator is contracting the upper lid upward (**Figs 7.2 & 7.3**).

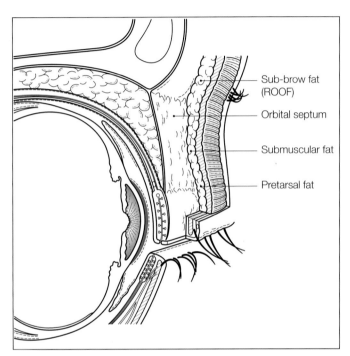

Sub-brow fat (ROOF)

Orbital septum

Submuscular fat

Pretarsal fat

Figure 7.2 Cross-sectional view of an Asian upper eyelid without lid crease. The orbital septum tends to fuse with the levator aponeurosis in a variable fashion from down over the anterior tarsal surface up to 5mm above the superior tarsal border. Besides the typical preaponeurotic (postseptal or orbital) fat pad, there is often presence of submuscular (suborbicularis oculi muscle, or preseptal) islands of fat pads, as well as pretarsal fat globules. The submuscular or preseptal fat may appear as an inferior extension of the sub-brow fat (or retro-orbicularis oculi fat). The upper tarsal plate measures from 6.5 to 8.0mm in Asians. (See Fig. 2.3.) (Reproduced with permission from Chen WP. Oculoplastic surgery: the essentials. New York: Thieme; 2001: 212.)

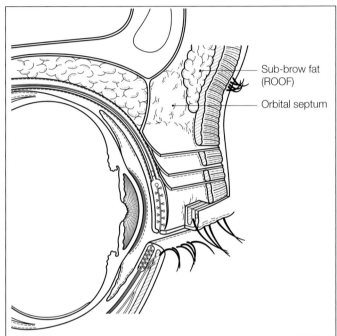

Sub-brow fat (ROOF)

Orbital septum

Figure 7.3 Cross-sectional view of a typical Caucasian eyelid with a natural upper eyelid crease. Aponeurotic fibers form interdigitations to the pretarsal orbicularis oculi muscle and a subdermal attachment along the superior tarsal border. The lid crease is often a composite of the vector forces from several of these creases. The pretarsal region is more anchored and firmer due to the presence of interdigitations of the terminal aponeurotic fibers. The orbital septum fuses with the levator aponeurosis at a higher level as compared with most Asians. There is less presence of the preaponeurotic fat inferiorly. There may be less submuscular fat as well as pretarsal fat. The upper tarsus is often 8.0–11.0mm in Caucasians. (Reproduced with permission from Chen WP. Oculoplastic surgery: the essentials. New York: Thieme; 2001: 212.)

The term 'westernizing blepharoplasty' is still quite often used to describe the crease procedure that Asians elect to undergo.[3] This can be complicating and misleading to the patient and physician alike. Such Asians really do not want to select the height and crease configuration of a Caucasian's or a Westerner's eye. Rather, most Asians who elect to have Asian blepharoplasty want to look like other Asians who have a crease – a very different crease as compared with that of a Caucasian.

Communication between patients and physicians is further weakened by additional confusion in terminology. The terms 'outer double eyelid' and 'inner double eyelid' do not refer to the higher crease found in a Caucasian (**Fig. 7.4**) versus the lower crease seen in those Asians who possess a crease, nor to any upslanting of the crease over the lateral canthus. Instead, they relate to the medial configuration (shape) of the crease among Asians. The term 'outer double' simply signifies a crease that does not converge to the medial canthus – I believe 'parallel' is a more appropriate term anatomically (**Fig. 7.5**). The term 'inner double eyelid' refers to a medially converging crease – I consider the term 'nasally tapered crease' is more accurate here (**Fig. 7.6**). The original terms make sense only if one appreciates the Chinese origin of these words, as they are English translations from Kanji (literal meaning: 'words of the Han race'), the language of the Han people. The abstract concepts are distorted in straight translation. Interestingly, the classical literature and Imperial court correspondences of Korean as well as Japanese cultures from the last 500 years both utilized Chinese Kanji. Overall, these terms are quite confusing for anyone who is not native to the Chinese written language. It is best to avoid using them for medicolegal reasons, since Chinese as well as non-Chinese Asians may be using them inaccurately.

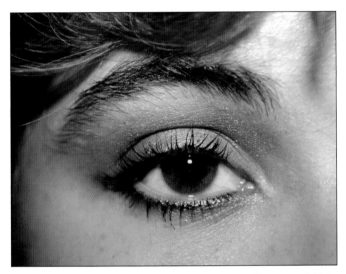

Figure 7.4 A typical semilunar crease for Caucasians. The crease is high by Asian norm and appears more separated from the lid margin over the central one-third of the eyelid.

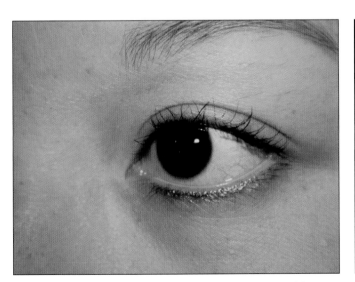

Figure 7.5 A parallel crease configuration. The crease runs equidistant from the lid margin as it courses from the medial to lateral canthus.

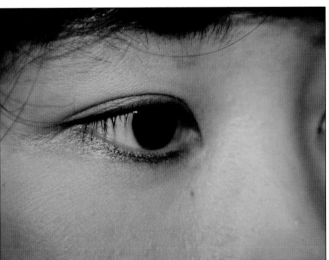

Figure 7.6 A nasally tapered crease configuration. The crease converges to the medial canthus and may either merge into it or stay converging but separated.

The term 'Asian blepharoplasty' was first used in a paper published in 1987 by this author.[1] The paper described a distinctive surgical procedure customized specifically for those Asians without a crease who desire to have a crease, and included details concerning the height and shape of such, and the surgical maneuvers needed to yield a crease that appears continuous, is predictable, and remains permanent in nature.

Through an external incision approach, the objective of Asian blepharoplasty is to clear a trapezoidal block of preaponeurotic tissues along the superior tarsal border, including the skin, orbicularis, orbital septum, as well as minimal preaponeurotic fat, in an equidepth and uniform fashion, to allow for optimal surgical apposition of the terminal fibers of the levator aponeurosis to the undersurface of the skin along the superior tarsal border.[4–7] For a nasally tapered crease, one would design the crease to converge medially. For a parallel crease, one would stay more level and equidistant along the lid margin.

Surgical method

The concept of upper eyelid crease configurations and the essential steps needed for predictable placement of a lid crease among those Asians without a crease have been covered in my previous publications.[1,4,5] My method is founded on accurate measurement of the central height of the upper tarsus, using it to determine the placement of the external incision line for creation of the crease. The ideal crease tends to be of either the nasally tapered type or of the parallel configuration. A medial upper lid fold is often present to some degree in the medial portion of the upper eyelid of Asians, whether they have a crease or not, and should not be considered pathologic, nor should it be automatically removed. Interestingly, the same small medial upper lid fold can be seen readily in non-Asians and even Europeans. (At present, the term 'epicanthal fold' seems to be indiscriminately applied to any degree of fold, no matter how small, and selectively applied to Asians, a practice I believe is unfortunate.)

Premedications and surgical setup

The patient usually receives 10mg of diazepam (Valium) and one tablet of Vicodin or Tylenol with codeine, orally, an hour before the procedure. The patient is placed in a supine position, and an intravenous line and electrocardiographic monitors are applied. A pulse oximeter that provides a real-time readout of the patient's pAO2 is applied. All patients are given a nasal cannula with 1–2L/min of room air flow (or oxygen). Intravenous Versed (midazolam) may be used in small aliquots of 0.5mg (0.5mL of 1mg/mL).

Anesthetic mixture and injections

Two mixtures of local anesthetics are then prepared:
1. 10mL of 2% lidocaine (Xylocaine) containing 1:100 000 dilution of epinephrine is mixed with 150 units of hyaluronidase*, if available, and labeled 'regular'. (This mixture is still acidic in nature.)
2. 1mL of the above mixture is further diluted with 9mL of injectable normal saline. This mixture now has a pH closer to neutrality since it has been diluted with the buffering action of injectable normal saline. The epinephrine concentration is now 1:1 000 000 (labeled 'diluted').

A drop of topical anesthetic, 0.5% proparacaine hydrochloride (Ophthaine, Ophthetic) is applied over each cornea for comfort prior to surgical preparation and draping. Using a 30-gauge half-inch needle, 0.25–0.5mL of the diluted mixture is infiltrated subcutaneously over the superior tarsal border of the mid-portion of the lid. During the next 2 minutes, anesthesia takes effect and one can observe blanching of the eyelid skin from the powerful vasoconstrictive effect of the diluted epinephrine (**Fig. 7.7**).

The regular mixture is then injected in the suborbicularis plane along the mid-section of the upper lid, usually applying less than 1.0mL per eyelid.

---

*Recently, the Pharmacy Services of the New England Compounding Center has begun to offer compounded hyaluronidase. (Telephone 800-994-6322, 697 Waverly Street, Framingham, MA 01702, USA.)

The purpose of this two-staged injection of local anesthetic is to allow for a relatively painless pre-infiltration to anesthetize the surgical field before the full strength of acidic 2% Xylocaine is given.[1] (One may add sodium bicarbonate to the 2% mix to achieve the same effect: for a 10% volume mixture, 1mL of 8.4% sodium bicarbonate, containing 100mEq or 8.4g per 100mL, is mixed with 9mL of the 2% Xylocaine.) The hyaluronidase promotes dispersion of the anesthetic and greatly reduces any tissue distortion, facilitating the identification of any crease line that the patient may have.

When confronted with a patient with a low threshold for pain, one may supplement the local field infiltration with a frontal nerve block: a 30-gauge half-inch needle may be used to apply 1mL of the anesthetic into the supraorbital space just lateral to the supraorbital notch.

The eyelids and face are then prepared in the usual fashion for ophthalmic plastic surgery. The eyes again receive a drop of topical anesthetic, this time using tetracaine hydrochloride for longer-lasting corneal anesthesia. To eliminate the possible sensation of claustrophobia that may occur with draping over the nose and midface, a single layer of sterile, moistened, porous gauze may be placed over the patient's exposed nose and mouth. Black opaque corneal protectors are then applied under the eyelids.

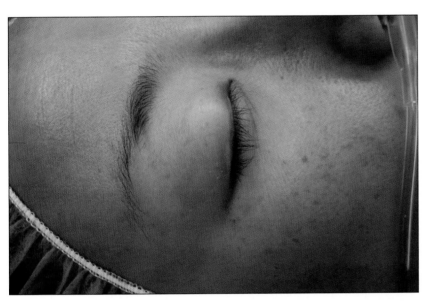

Figure 7.7 Blanching of skin following injection of anesthetic mixture containing diluted epinephrine. Intense vasoconstriction is seen even with dilution of 1:1 000 000 epinephrine.

 Clinical pearls

- The use of diluted anesthetic solution helps to:
  - decrease pain upon injection;
  - decrease volume of anesthetic needed for injection; and
  - create less tissue distortion as a result of less volume expansion and lessened bleeding.
- It allows the surgeon to stay focused on the surgical plane.
- The use of nasally delivered room air or low-flow oxygen serves to decrease the patient's sense of claustrophobia.

Pitfalls

- Never use nasal oxygen in an open system exposed to monopolar cautery, as it may cause ignition and flaming.
- Always apply pulse oximetry to measure the pAO2 saturation. Preoperative sedation and intraoperative sedation may easily cause apnea in a sensitive patient.

Surgical stages

The height of the tarsus determines the overall central position of the surgical crease; the shape is determined by how you design the medial one-third and lateral one-third of this lower line of incision, according to the patient's preference.

The shaved-off tip of a wooden cotton-tip applicator dipped with methylene blue is used to indicate the proposed crease. The upper lid is everted and the vertical height of the tarsus is measured over the central portion of the lid with a caliper (**Fig. 7.8**). This measurement – which is usually between 6.5 and 8.0mm – is carefully transcribed onto the external skin surface, again over the central part of the eyelid skin. This point directly overlies the superior tarsal border and will serve as a reference point for the overall crease *height* along the *central* one-third of the eyelid, whether the crease *shape* is to be nasally tapered, parallel, or, in rare cases, laterally flared. For those patients who have a crease, one should also measure the tarsus to confirm that the apparent crease is indeed the correct crease line to use, whether one is planning to preserve or enhance it.

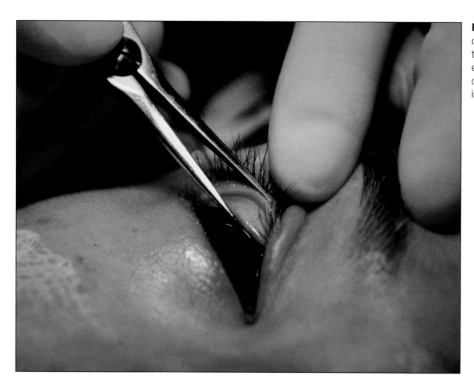

Figure 7.8 The upper eyelid is everted and a caliper used to measure the central height of the tarsus. This point is transcribed onto the external surface of the skin and serves as a central reference point for the lower line of incision.

If the crease is to be nasally tapered, with either a laterally leveled or flared configuration, the *medial* one-third of the incision line is marked such that it tapers towards the medial canthal angle or merges with the medial upper lid fold (**Fig. 7.9**). The *lateral* one-third is usually marked in a leveled configuration, although occasionally a patient may request a slight upward widening over the lateral segment of the crease.

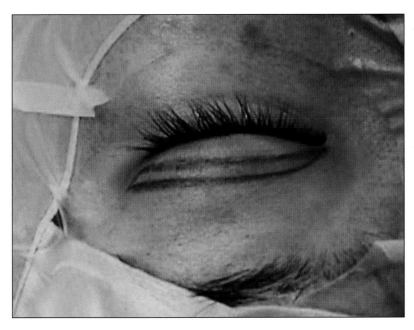

Figure 7.9 Marking and design of a nasally tapered crease. The medial one-third of the incision lines taper towards the medial canthal angle. The lateral one-third may be either leveled or flared upward.

Clinical pearls

■ The use of an inked tapered tip of a wooden stick allows precise drawing and redrawing, as compared with the usual marking-pen available in operating theaters.

■ In Asian blepharoplasty involving skin excision, the lower line of incision will determine the shape and height of the surgically created crease.

■ Repetitive measurement and confirmation of incision lines are important.

■ Usually, 1–3mm of skin may be included in the incision line for excision.

■ Using the thinned wooden-tip applicator and applying very gentle pressure on the lower incision line (proposed line for new crease formation), instruct the patient to look upward even before the incision starts, in order to assess how the crease may appear. Since the eyelid has been injected, the crease will appear more swollen and further from the ciliary margin than it will postoperatively, after it has eventually healed.

For the parallel crease, the measured height of the superior tarsal border is drawn across the width of the eyelid skin (**Fig. 7.10**).

To create adequate adhesions, some subdermal tissue must be removed. A strip of skin measuring about 2mm is then marked above and parallel to this *lower* line of incision. In patients who want a nasally tapered configuration, this *upper* line of incision is tapered towards the medial canthal angle, or to merge with any medial upper lid fold that may be present. The segment of skin to be excised is frequently less than 2mm over the medial portion of the crease.

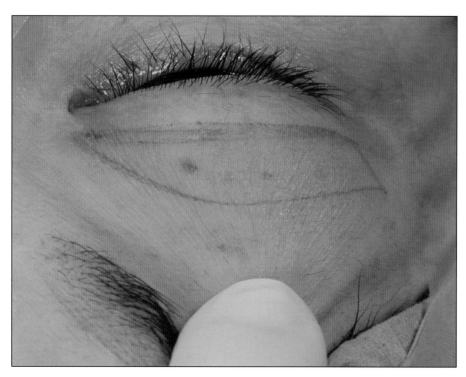

Figure 7.10 Marking and design of a parallel crease.

Clinical pearls

- In designing the parallel crease, there is an unconscious tendency to converge towards the medial canthal angle, thereby turning it into a nasally tapered crease. I often intentionally draw the tapering crease first and then use it as a visual guide to decide how a parallel crease should be designed near the medial one-third of the upper lid, to remind myself to stay parallel.

Pitfalls

- Medially, the parallel crease does not flare upward from the medial canthal angle.

- The medial end of the crease design should not go past an imaginary vertical line aligned with the medial canthal angle, both for nasally tapered and for parallel creases.

- Laterally, the crease design should not traverse past the lateral canthal angle.

The incision is then carried out using a No. 15 surgical blade (Bard-Parker) along the upper and lower lines, incising just through the dermis and within the superficial orbicularis oculi muscles. Fine capillary bleeding is controlled using bipolar wetfield cautery (**Fig. 7.11**).

The excision of a strip of skin is not required in every case; however, I believe that it facilitates the removal of subsequent layers of the lid tissues, thereby permitting adequate crease formation. At this point, the superior tarsal border is still covered by pretarsal and supratarsal* (favored over the term 'preseptal') orbicularis oculi muscle, with possibly some terminal portions of the orbital septum, and the terminal fibers of the levator aponeurosis beneath the septum.

---

*Semantically, in Asians, the supratarsal area is an area directly above the tarsus, while the true preseptal region may be quite a few millimeters superior to this, since the orbital septum may fuse with the levator aponeurosis a variable distance from the superior tarsal border.

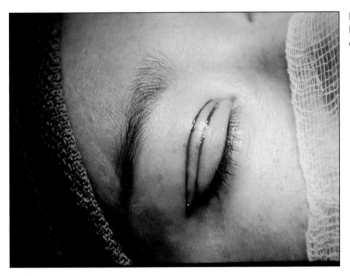

Figure 7.11 Upper and lower lines of incision have been opened with a No. 15 surgical blade, with wetfield bipolar cautery applied to vascular oozing that may arise from orbicularis muscle.

Clinical pearls

■ It is important to stabilize the tarsal plate and overlying soft tissues and skin when making a continuous incision, especially along the lower line of incision; this is a critical step in the outcome of the designed crease.

■ The continuous incision may be performed in three steps so that one may check and recheck the passage. For right-handed surgeons, for the right upper lid, it is best to start medially; and for the left upper lid, one may start from the lateral end of the incision line.

■ Any bleeding is best controlled with bipolar cautery via a fine jeweler's tip. This allows the surgeon to lessen any immediate tissue swelling and obscuration of the tissue planes, thereby maintaining a clear operative field. Furthermore, it allows one to stay within the planned incision line.

Pitfalls

■ It is easy to incise too deeply and cause a small steady bleed from the orbicularis muscle, which will soon develop into a hematoma and distort the incision line as well as incision planes, blurring the distinction between fat, orbicularis, orbital septum, and levator aponeurosis along the superior tarsal border. It may also result in transient postoperative secondary ptosis.

One may use the left fingers to slightly retract the upper incision wound edge, then aim a Bovie cautery tip (or radiofrequency unit's Empire tip needle) superiorly to transect through the preseptal orbicularis oculi muscle there, knowing that although the upper incision line is only 2–3mm above the superior tarsal border, with the upward beveling, the Bovie tip is aiming at a point above where the septum fuses with the aponeurosis. (In Asians, the orbital septum may join the aponeurosis as low as 2–3mm above the superior tarsal border.) The use of the cutting cautery tip is in a feather-light fashion, so as to gently reach the orbital septum. Along the way, one may see some preseptal fat in front of the septum. When the septum over the central one-third is opened, one can see the slightly bulging preaponeurotic fat pad prolapsing through the opening of the orbital septum (**Fig. 7.12**). Blunt-tipped Westcott's spring scissors are then used to open the orbital septum.

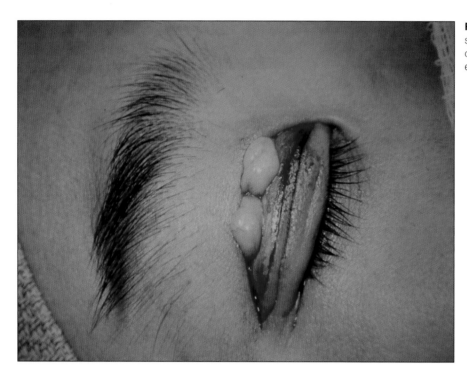

Figure 7.12 After traversing through the supratarsal orbicularis in a beveled fashion, the orbital septum is reached and opened horizontally, exposing the underlying preaponeurotic fat pads.

 Clinical pearls

- Always tilt the tips of the scissors upward when extending the horizontal release of the orbital septum to either side. The purpose is to avoid inadvertent injury to the vessels within the fat pad, the fat pad itself, the underlying levator aponeurosis, or the lobe of the lacrimal gland situated over the lateral end.

 Pitfalls

- In opening of the orbital septum medially, the levator aponeurosis may be injured.

- In opening of the lateral extent of the septum, the lacimal gland can be injured.

- Avoid the use of monopolar cautery over the superior medial aspect of the orbital space to avoid the trochlea of the superior oblique muscle, which can lead to fourth-nerve palsy and torsional diplopia.

- Avoid cauterizing the lacrimal gland over the superior lateral aspect of the anterior orbital rim.

The orbital septum is opened along the superior line of incision and the skin–orbicularis–orbital septum flap turned inferiorly along the superior tarsal border (**Fig. 7.13**).

Westcott scissors are used to open the potential space that is present between the preaponeurotic fat and the overlying orbicularis muscle within the redundant myocutaneous strip, retracting it with a Blair's tissue retractor. The central preaponeurotic fat pad is dissected and separated from its fascial attachment to its underlying levator muscle fibers (it is salmon-colored with vertically oriented muscle striations).

The fat should be repositioned, allowing it to fill in the space between the levator and anterior aspect of the superior orbital rim (the supratarsal sulcus).

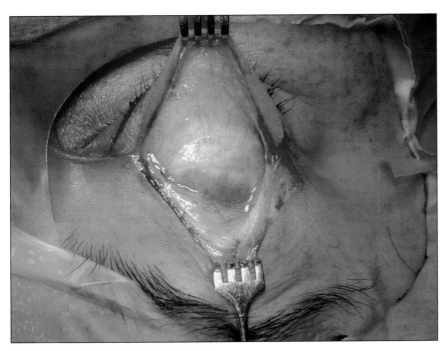

Figure 7.13 The skin–orbicularis–septal flap may be rotated inferiorly to facilitate exposure to the preaponeurotic fat pads and the underlying levator aponeurosis.

Clinical pearls

- After separating the initial fine adhesions of fat from the overlying orbicularis, it is often safer to use moist cotton-tip applicators to separate fat from the underlying superior tarsal border, levator aponeurosis, and levator muscle.

- No attempt is made to remove the fat pad unless it is grossly interfering with crease formation along the superior tarsal border. Wetfield bipolar cautery may be used to shrink it away if it is potentially 'threatening' the construction of a good crease because of its presence directly over the preaponeurotic platform.

Pitfalls

- Avoid pointing the scissors posteriorly towards the levator as you elevate the myocutaneous flap.

- After the myocutaneous flap has been elevated, avoid cutting any fat that may be intertwined on the underbelly of the myocutaneous strip; this may cause bleeding of the intra-fat blood vessels, as well as inadvertent reduction in the volume of preaponeurotic fat left behind.

Occasionally, in patients with very full upper lids, significant fat is seen centrally and in an inferiorly placed position. This may significantly abort/interfere with any attempt to form a crease. In these patients, instead of mild reduction with bipolar cautery, one may opt to excise 25–50% of the preaponeurotic fat seen within the surgical field (**Fig. 7.14**). Wetfield cautery is used to treat the intra-fat vessels first; then cutting monopolar cautery is used to cut the fat pad 2–3mm at a time. These maneuvers are then repeated. It may take two to three repetitions before this stage is completed. (The fat excision often necessitates a small supplement of lidocaine in the space underneath the preaponeurotic fat pad.)

If a patient with dermatochalasis and obliteration of crease should manifest even a very minimal concavity in the supratarsal sulcus, one should not remove any fat, as this will worsen the hollowness and cause multiple redundant folds superior to where one wants the crease to be. Instead of excision of the fat, one should reposition it above.

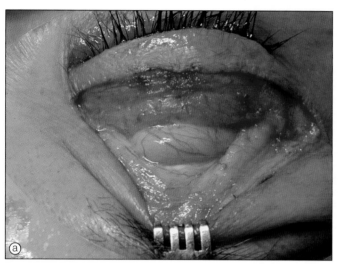
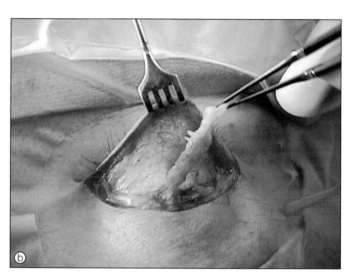

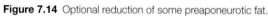
Figure 7.14 Optional reduction of some preaponeurotic fat.

Clinical pearls

- Extra care and time is allotted to this step of reduction of fat pads, if elected. Hemorrhage from undetected bleeders following transection of the intra-fat vessels may lead to serious consequences, including orbital hematoma and blindness.

- A prolapsed lacrimal gland may look like a lobe of fat. It must be recognized and needs to be reanchored to a point behind the superior-lateral orbital rim (see Chapter 5).

Pitfalls

- It is important to clearly distinguish the nasal fat pad and central preaponeurotic fat pad from the lacrimal gland lobule.

- Transection of the lacrimal gland may lead to varying degrees of dry eyes.

Figure 7.15 shows excision of the myocutaneous flap (skin, orbicularis, and inferior remnants of septum) along the superior tarsal border. This is carried out by grasping the lateral end of the myocutaneous flap of the right upper lid (or medial end of the left upper lid myocutaneous flap) with the instrument in your left hand, then using the radiofrequency unit or monopolar needle tip on cutting mode to cut along a plane between the orbicularis within the flap and the superior tarsal border/aponeurotic junction.

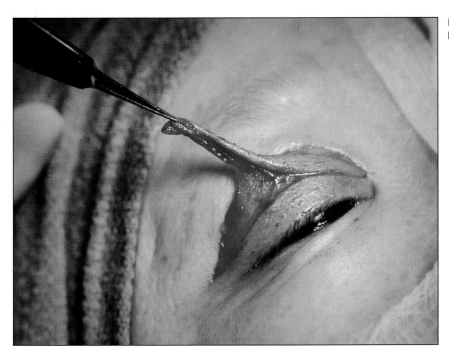

Figure 7.15 The myocutaneous flap is then trimmed horizontally along the superior tarsal border.

 Clinical pearls

■ When the myocutaneous flap is incised, the orbicularis muscle will bleed. As one proceeds, one should control each of the new bleeders as soon as they arise, using bipolar cautery, rather than cutting off the whole strip first, before coming back to control a group of bleeders. This seems to decrease postoperative edema and hematoma formation.

■ There is a tendency to go too shallow over the medial starting point of the left upper lid during this phase of the excision of the myocutaneous strip, leaving behind too much orbicularis. An inadequately anchored crease over the medial segment may therefore result from this subtle oversight.

 Pitfalls

■ One must take care to avoid inadvertent partial transection of the distal fibers of the levator aponeurosis.

■ Avoid transection of the superior tarsal vascular arcade, which may bleed and cause segmental swelling and postoperative secondary ptosis.

Figure 7.16 represents a three-dimensional line drawing of trapezoidal debulking of the preaponeurotic platform.

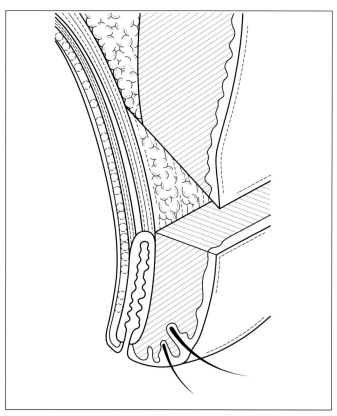

Figure 7.16 Cross-sectional drawing of trapezoidal debulking of the preaponeurotic platform in Asian blepharoplasty.

Clinical pearls

- This trapezoidal 'one-plane' debulking of the preaponeurotic platform is an efficient, elegant, and controlled technique of excising a whole block of redundant tissues, with full control of tissues excised in an equi-depth fashion.

- The beveled plane allows the tissues to appose nicely during surgical closure.

- Instruct the patient to look up, to evaluate your attempt at crease formation. Any incomplete formation of crease should be investigated at this point.

After excision of the myocutaneous strip, often there is some residual fascial tissue along the lower skin incision wound. This is composed of a combination of preseptal and pretarsal orbicularis muscle fibers, interspersed with occasional pretarsal fat patches. This may occupy the path along which one is planning to form the crease, just over the superior tarsal border. In this situation, it is advisable to excise this 2–3mm strip of orbicularis tissues along the inferior skin incision edge (**Fig. 7.17**). It allows a smoothing and mild flattening of the tissues along the pretarsal plane, as well as thinning of the inferior wound edge.

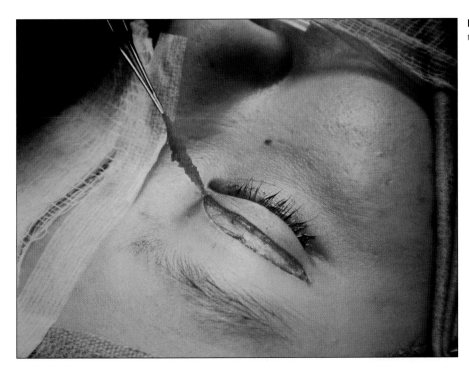

Figure 7.17 A strip of pretarsal orbicularis muscle is trimmed along the lower skin incision.

 Clinical pearls

■ The pretarsal tissue may be reduced only if pretarsal fat is moderately abundant and threatens the surgical formation of the desired upper lid crease.

■ There are some authors who routinely debulk the entire pretarsal subcutaneous tissue, believing that it is better to have only skin over the anterior surface of the tarsus. This may come about because of concerns that there are competing distal fibers of the levator aponeurosis within the pretarsal plane. In reality, within the pretarsal plane of a creaseless Asian eyelid, there are few, if any, functional terminal interdigitations of the levator aponeurosis to the dermis.

 Pitfalls

■ Vigorous dissection along the pretarsal plane is not advisable as it creates prolonged postoperative edema and can risk undesirable formation of multiple creases. Furthermore, it is quite normal for Asians born with a natural crease to have some degree of pretarsal fullness along the area between the crease and the eyelashes.

■ Leaving behind redundant tissues along the inferior border may result in only partial formation of the crease or late obliteration of an initially acceptable crease.

The adhesive surgical drapes over the patient's mid-forehead and upper eyelid skin are then loosened, to decrease any upward traction over the incision wound, tarsus, and eyelid margin.

In order to form a dynamic crease*, the terminal fibers of the levator aponeurosis above the superior tarsal border should be directed to the subdermal plane of the lower line of skin incision. 6-0 nonabsorbable suture (6-0 silk or nylon) is used to pick up the lower skin edge and subcutaneous tissue, the levator aponeurosis along the superior tarsal border, and then the upper skin edge. Each of these is tied as an interrupted suture.

Besides the stitch over the center of the crease, three interrupted sutures are placed medially and two to three stitches laterally. With these six to seven crease-forming sutures in place, the rest of the incision may be closed using 6-0 or 7-0 silk/nylon in a continuous or subcuticular fashion (**Fig. 7.18a**). This gives the best chance for the formation of a dynamic crease.

Some surgeons prefer to bury either dissolvable or permanent stitches along the superior tarsal border, fixating the inferior edge of the pretarsal orbicularis to the levator muscle. This method, in my experience, tends to give a static crease. Some patients complain of persistent foreign body sensation within the muscle layers of the lid many years after buried permanent sutures have been applied. These often have to be removed secondarily.

---

*A dynamic crease of the upper eyelid is a surgically created crease that fades on downgaze. A static crease remains obvious on downgaze.

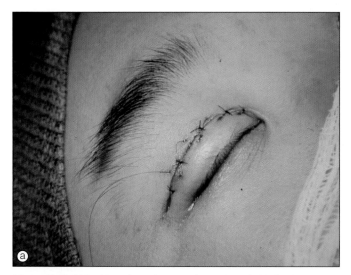
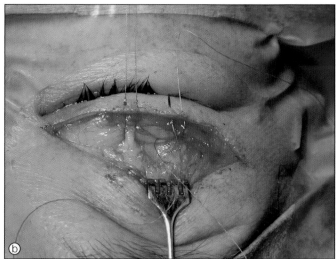

Figure 7.18 (a) In this patient, the wound was closed with five interrupted 6-0 sutures and a continuous 7-0 nylon suture. (b) Crease fixation sutures using Vicryl sutures, applying them from pretarsal skin to levator aponeurosis along the superior tarsal border.

Clinical pearls

- The medial end of the crease may require additional placement of crease-forming (skin/levator/skin) sutures, as the medial extent of the levator muscle is often rudimentary and underdeveloped.

- In a patient with a medial canthal fold, if a nasally tapered crease shape was preselected, the crease line can often be designed to merge medially into the fold itself.

- In applying the crease-forming stitch, each bite on the aponeurosis should be at the superior tarsal border and not any higher, to prevent the formation of a 'high, harsh and semilunar crease'.

- To enhance or deepen a crease, one may apply three double-armed 5-0 Vicryl sutures transcutaneously to the underlying tarsus along the superior tarsal border (locating these over the medial, central, and lateral one-thirds of the eyelid) just below the crease line, in addition to the skin closure (**Fig. 7.18b**). The sutures are then tied externally. After 1 week, the knot is trimmed off the skin, leaving behind the buried loop of the absorbable Vicryl.

- Check crease symmetry bilaterally upon completion of closure. Measure the crease height with a caliper. If there is a discrepancy, it is better to correct the difference in crease height between the two sides by revising the higher crease down, through excision of 0.5–1.0mm of skin from the inferior skin edge of this side. This is a general rule and should be applied only with individual evaluation.

 Pitfalls

- One is likely to end up with upper eyelid retraction or secondary ectropion if the tissues have not been allowed to lay back to their natural plane prior to surgical closure.

- Insufficient inclusion of the levator aponeurosis will result in partial crease formation or late obliteration.

- Excessively deep or high bite along the levator aponeurosis may result in a high crease or an acquired secondary ptosis, with secondary lagophthalomos on upgaze.

- Patients who manifest ptosis will tend to have poor crease formation. It is best to address the ptosis repair first and return later to create a crease.

- Inclusion of residual fat pads along the superior tarsal border will result in obliteration of crease.

Postoperative Regimen for Asian Blepharoplasty Patients

- Ice compresses for 1 day.

- Bed rest for 24 hours.

- No reading, viewing of television, or computer use. No computer-gaming.

- Wound and facial hygiene – clean face and incision wounds three to four times daily with clean water.

- Apply antibiotic ointment four times daily for 7 days.

- Patient may shower that day.

- Avoid hot-spa or swimming.

- Avoid strenuous activities or workout for at least a week.

- Avoid aspirin compounds or anything with ibuprofen (Moltin). Steroids are not routinely prescribed.

- Avoid consumption of spicy foods, chocolate, dairy products, and fried foods for 2 months.

Patients without any pre-existing crease should undertake the following crease-enhancing eye version exercise. Patients are instructed to try looking upward (actuation of the levator function) from the third postoperative day onward. The patient is taught to assume a normal, vertically aligned frontal-to-chin head posture and refrain from using the frontalis muscle of the forehead, then to look from a downgaze to an upward position, at least ten repetitions, twice a day. The speed of levator movement should be deliberately slow in order to allow good crease in-folding without pulling on any fine blood vessels and causing postoperative hematoma.

Suture removal is at 1 week.

The patients are told that 80% of the postoperative swelling should disappear a week after the sutures have been removed or at 2 weeks postoperatively. The remaining swelling may linger for 2 months. They are instructed that the crease may change over a period of 9–12 months.

Should there be a need for revision touch-up – for example, when the crease did not form distinctively – the touch-up is performed no earlier than 6 months, as the crease continues to mature. This author does not advocate secondary revision on patients seeking consultation after having had previous procedure(s) elsewhere unless a 12-month period has elapsed.

Some preoperative photos and postoperative results are shown in **Figures 7.19–7.30**.

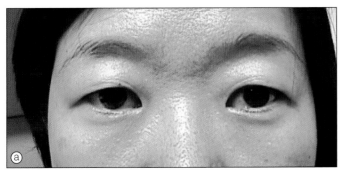
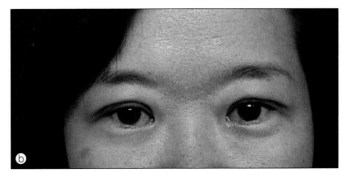

Figure 7.19 (a) Before and (b) after.

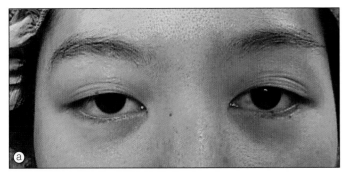
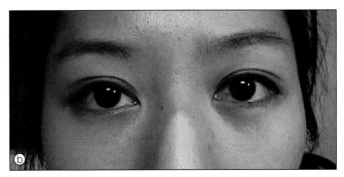

Figure 7.20 (a) Before and (b) after.

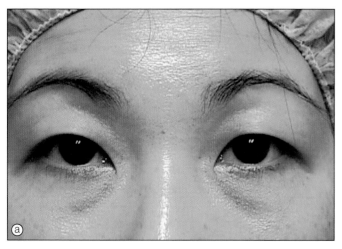

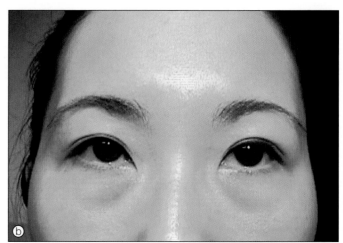

Figure 7.21 (a) Before and (b) after.

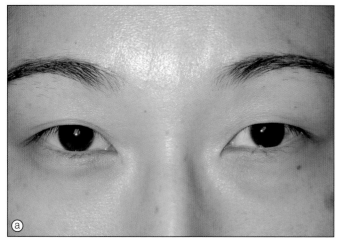

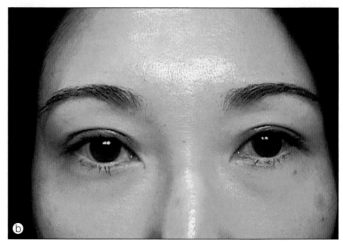

Figure 7.22 (a) Before and (b) after.

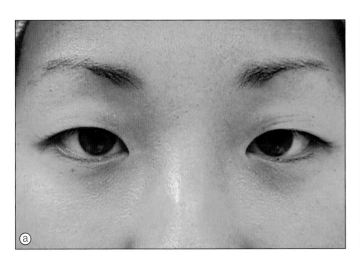

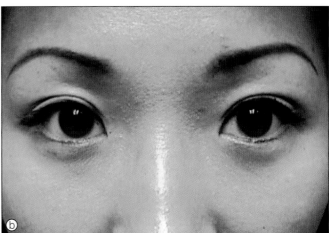

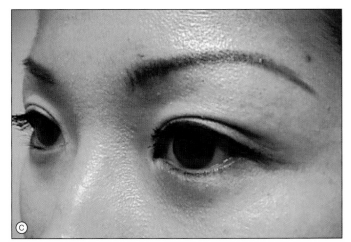

Figure 7.23 (a) Before, (b) after and (c) after - oblique view.

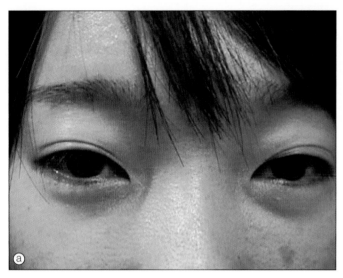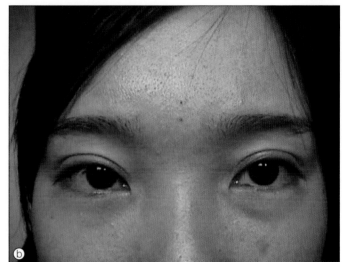

Figure 7.24 (a) Before and (b) after.

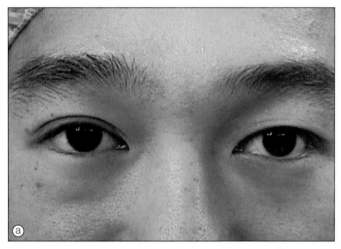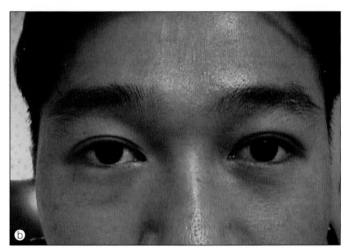

Figure 7.25 (a) Before and (b) after.

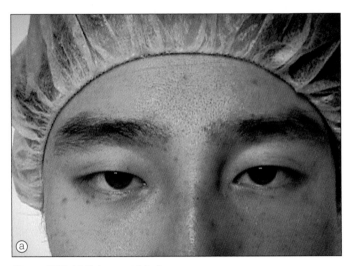
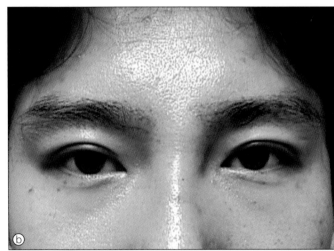

Figure 7.26 (a) Before and (b) after.

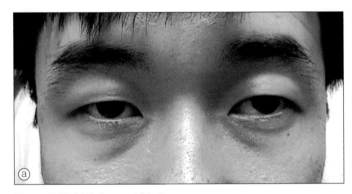
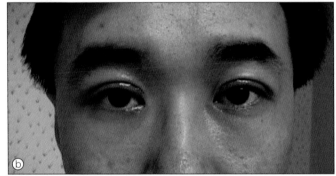

Figure 7.27 (a) Before and (b) after.

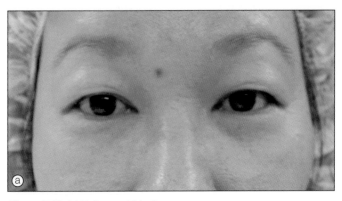
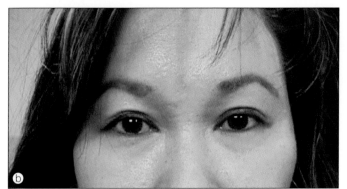

Figure 7.28 (a) Before and (b) after.

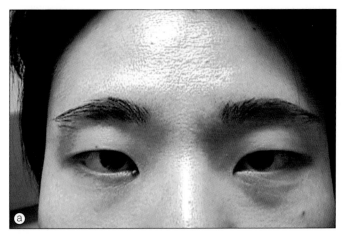
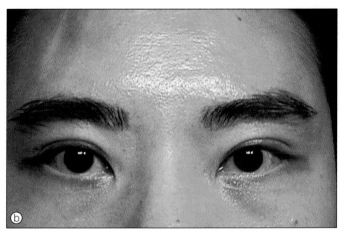

Figure 7.29 (a) Before and (b) after.

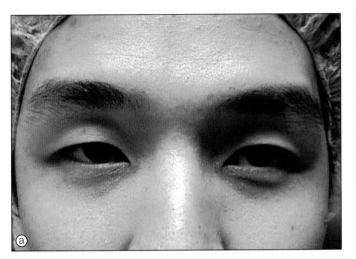

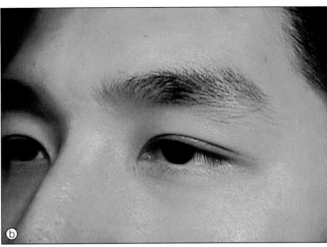

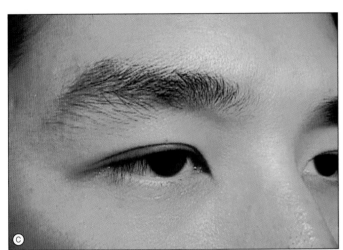

Figure 7.30 (a) Before and (b, c) after.

Clinical Use

Elderly Asian patients, with or without a pre-existing upper lid crease, may present with:

- dermatochalasis alone (**Fig. 7.31**);

- dermatochalasis with fatty prolapse; or

- dermatochalasis with ptosis (**Fig. 7.32**).

Surgical solutions for such are as follows (**Fig. 7.33**):

1. *Elderly Asian patients with a pre-existing crease*

- Dermatochalasis alone is corrected by preserving the crease, and carrying out a skin-excision blepharoplasty.

- Dermatochalasis with fatty prolapse is best managed by preserving the crease, and performing a blepharoplasty with trimming of only sufficient fat above the superior tarsal border to permit preservation of the crease. (Excess fat excision will result in deepening of the supratarsal sulcus.)

- In dermatochalasis with ptosis, the crease has often migrated upward; the crease should be reset based on the individual's tarsal height using Asian blepharoplasty, performing only skin excision plus levator aponeurotic repair (resection and/or advancement).

2. *Elderly Asian patients without a pre-existing crease*

These patients can opt to have a crease added.

- Dermatochalasis alone is corrected by Asian blepharoplasty with excision of the dermatochalasis and creation of a lid crease (if the patient wants one).

- Dermatochalasis with fatty prolapse is corrected by Asian blepharoplasty with excision of the dermatochalasis and creation of a lid crease (if the patient wants one), with trimming of only sufficient fat to permit making of a crease.

- Dermatochalasis with ptosis is rectified using skin-excision-only Asian blepharoplasty, with creation of a lid crease, plus levator aponeurotic repair (resection and/or advancement).

When the elderly Asian patient does not have a pre-existing crease and prefers to stay crease-less:

- Dermatochalasis alone is corrected by skin excision blepharoplasty and closure without crease fixation.

- Dermatochalasis with fatty prolapse is corrected by skin excision blepharoplasty, minimal fat excision, and closure without crease fixation.

- Dermatochalasis with ptosis is corrected by skin excision blepharoplasty plus levator aponeurotic repair (resection and/or advancement), and closure without crease fixation.

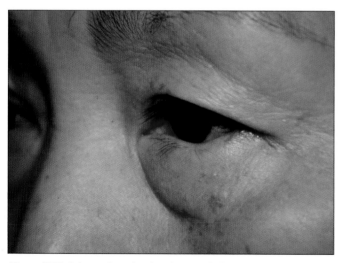

Figure 7.31 Asian patient showing dermatochalasis of the upper eyelid.

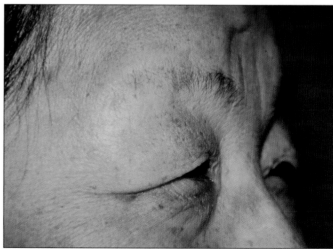

Figure 7.32 Asian patient showing dermatochalasis and ptosis.

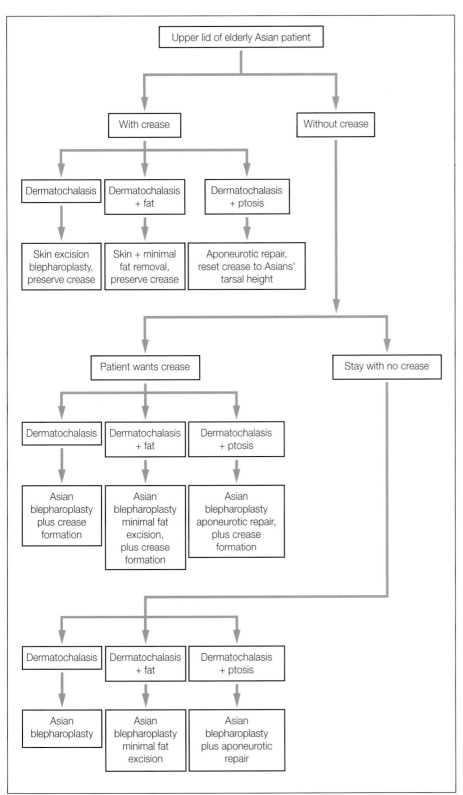

Figure 7.33 Surgical solutions for Asian blepharoplasty in elderly patients. (Reproduced with permission from Chen WP. Oculoplastic surgery: the essentials. New York: Thieme; 2001: 221.)

The Suture Ligation Method

There are alternatives to the external incision method of the double eyelid crease procedure, one of which is using suture ligation alone without extensive incision and excision. The surgical objective of the ligation (suturing) approach is to create a surgical adhesion between the soft tissues just above the tarsal plate to the overlying skin, whether the surgical ligature is first inserted through the conjunctival side or from the skin side, and whether it is ligated with the suture knot buried under the subconjunctival side or the subcutaneous side. The key element is a lack of tissue removal and this is also a limitation. There are usually three to five stitches used among variations of this method. The method does not involve any extensive relayering, excision, or removal of soft tissue, and so will not correct for any anatomic soft tissue redundancy. It works relatively well for young adults aged up to early 20s. Beyond this age group, the natural increase in soft tissue mass over the preaponeurotic platform, whether due to aging or to gravitational sagging, renders the suture ligation method less effective. Satisfaction levels, short term, seem high among patients in Japan. If a patient is willing to consider a crease that may vanish or be shielded-over from view after 2 to 10 years, and is willing to undergo repeat surgery, this is an alternative. Patients' complaints may include persistent foreign body sensation, irregularity in the contour of the crease (e.g. 'bamboo-like' truncation of segments of the crease), unevenness in the depth of the crease in the medial, central, or lateral third of the eyelid, granuloma formation, and 'static' appearance of the crease on downgaze.

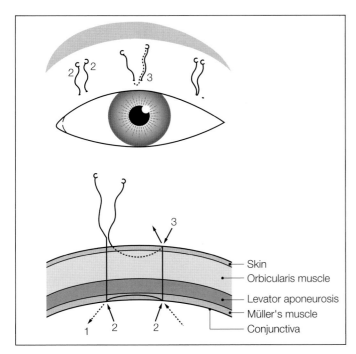

Figure 7.34 Full-thickness suturing technique. (Reproduced with permission from Chen WPD. Asian blepharoplasty: a surgical atlas. Newton: Butterworth and Heinemann; 1995: 38.)

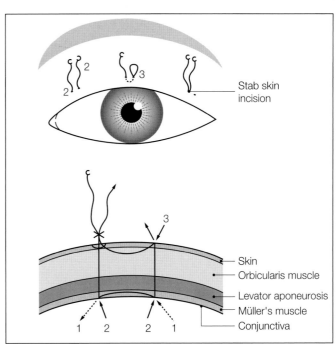

Figure 7.35 Full-thickness suturing technique with stab incisions. (Reproduced with permission from Chen WPD. Asian blepharoplasty: a surgical atlas. Newton: Butterworth and Heinemann; 1995: 39.)

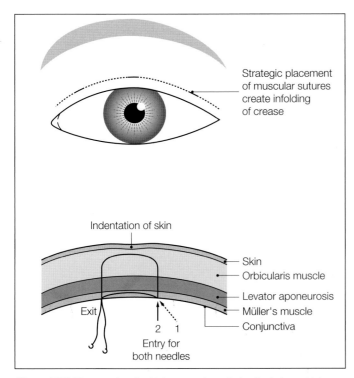

Figure 7.36 Transconjunctival intramuscular suturing technique. Note the absence of passage through skin. (Reproduced with permission from Chen WPD. Asian blepharoplasty: a surgical atlas. Newton: Butterworth and Heinemann; 1995: 40.)

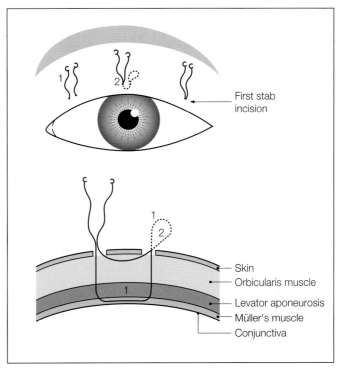

Figure 7.37 Transcutaneous intramuscular suturing technique. (Reproduced with permission from Chen WPD. Asian blepharoplasty: a surgical atlas. Newton: Butterworth and Heinemann; 1995: 41.)

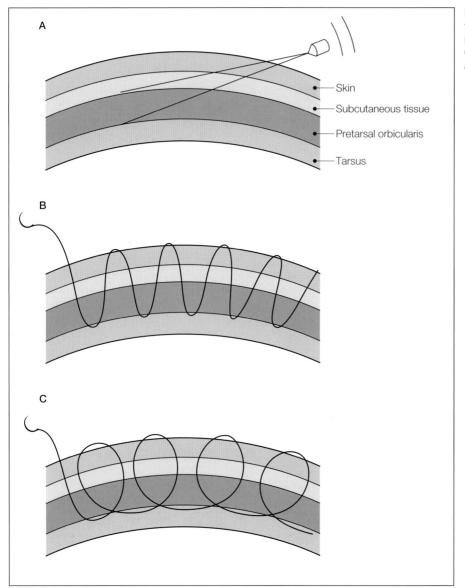

A

Skin
Subcutaneous tissue
Pretarsal orbicularis
Tarsus

B

C

Figure 7.38 Twisted needle and compression technique with transcutaneous intratarsal suturing. (Reproduced with permission from Chen WPD. Asian blepharoplasty: a surgical atlas. Newton: Butterworth and Heinemann; 1995: 42.)

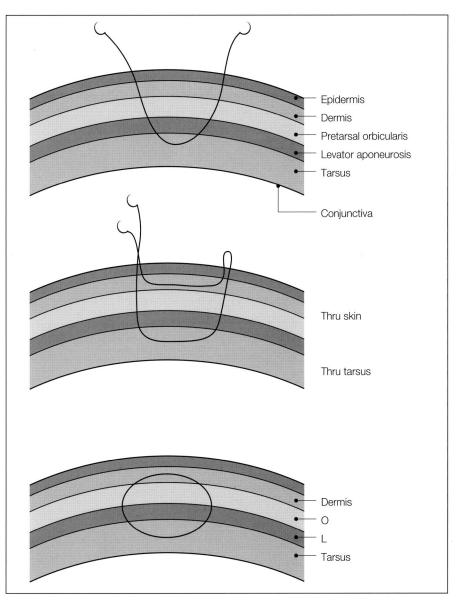

Epidermis
Dermis
Pretarsal orbicularis
Levator aponeurosis
Tarsus

Conjunctiva

Thru skin

Thru tarsus

Dermis
O
L
Tarsus

Figure 7.39 Transcutaneous intradermal and intratarsal suturing technique. L, levator aponeurosis; O, orbicularis. (Reproduced with permission from Chen WPD. Asian blepharoplasty: a surgical atlas. Newton: Butterworth and Heinemann; 1995: 39.)

The Advanced Concept of Triangular, Trapezoidal, and Rectangular Debulking of Eyelid Tissues, as Applied in Asian Blepharoplasty

In the past, double eyelid procedures were carried out through various external incision methods, which may have involved removing skin,[8] skin with orbicularis,[9,10] skin with pretarsal fat,[11] or excision of skin, muscle, orbital septum, and preaponeurotic fat.[12,13] They were all attempts at creating a clear platform for the formation of adhesions between fibers of the levator aponeurosis and the subcutaneous structure of the surgically created crease. However, because the excision may not be uniformly carried out over the width of the crease, often an irregular platform of tissues anterior to the superior tarsal border is left behind and this will interfere with the definition and formation of the crease.

The author's method[4] of triangular and trapezoidal debulking allows a systematic and uniform cleaning of the preaponeurotic platform over and along the superior tarsal border. As **Figure 7.40** shows:

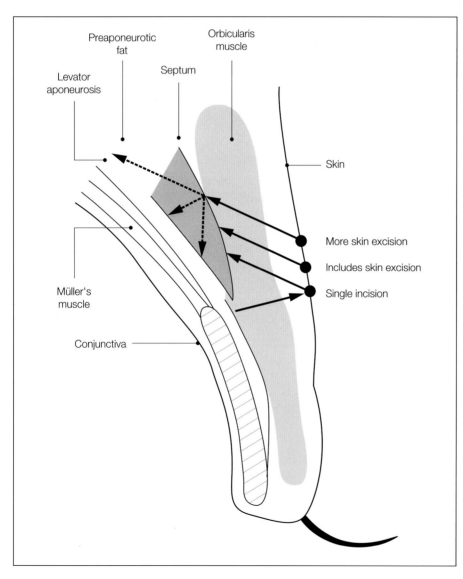

Figure 7.40 Cross-sectional drawing of an Asian upper eyelid without upper lid crease. Black dots correspond to lines of skin incision. Solid arrows correspond to the transorbicularis vector from skin to orbital septum. Dotted arrows show possible plane of dissection through the preaponeurotic fat pads. Trapezoidal debulking of preaponeurotic tissues in Asian blepharoplasty may include all tissues bounded by the upper and lower transorbicularis vectors, and that between the skin and the orbital septum. Minimal fat excision may also be included. (Reproduced with permission from Chen WPD. Asian blepharoplasty: a surgical atlas. Newton: Butterworth and Heinemann; 1995: 165.)

1. When skin excision (<2mm) is performed in conjunction with placement of the lid crease, retracting the upper skin incision edge permits an upwardly beveled plane of dissection to proceed across the supratarsal orbicularis oculi muscle and the lower portion of the orbital septum. (In Asians without a crease in the upper lid, the orbital septum is often fused to the levator aponeurosis at 2–4mm above the superior tarsal border, and it can be as low as halfway down the anterior surface of the tarsus.) The septum and underlying preaponeurotic fat pads may be easily identified.

2. The septum orbitale is opened horizontally. This *trapezoid* (viewed in cross-section) of preaponeurotic tissues, including sometimes a minimal amount of preaponeurotic fat, the orbital septum, supratarsal orbicularis, subcutaneous fat, and overlying skin (<2mm), all of which hinges along the superior tarsal border, may be debulked. The anterior surface of this conceptual trapezoid consists of the skin, while the posterior portion of the trapezoid is wider and includes all preaponeurotic tissues from the opened orbital septum down to the superior tarsal border.

3. A small strand of the pretarsal orbicularis along the inferior skin incision may be trimmed off.

4. The trapezoidal debulking allows simple inward folding of the skin edges towards the underlying aponeurosis, facilitating the surgical formation of the crease. (The microscopic study by Collin et al.[2] described insertions of distal strands of the levator aponeurosis into the septa in between pretarsal orbicularis oculi muscle fibers, rather than into any subdermal tissue along the lid crease in those eyelids that had crease. If true, formation of a crease may be facilitated by the above surgical maneuver, as it links the aponeurosis to the upper border of the pretarsal zone.) Vigorous dissection and debulking of pretarsal tissues is to be avoided for reasons mentioned previously.

When debulking is carried out without including any skin excision, the block of tissue removed will resemble a *triangular* configuration in cross-sectional view.

Should there be significant skin redundancy, the amount of skin included for excision is increased by moving up the upper line of skin incision. The plane of dissection through the orbicularis then becomes less beveled and the *trapezoidal* debulking gradually transforms into more of a *rectangular* configuration.

Figure 7.41 shows the transorbicularis vector (Step 2) for the dissection plane rotating counter-clockwise and leveling off as one takes away more skin and the upper line of skin incision – 1(U) – moves further away from the superior tarsal border (level of STB).

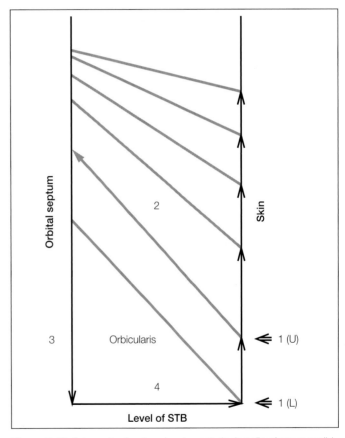

Figure 7.41 Schematic drawing showing anterior lamella of upper eyelid, with orbicularis of the supratarsal region and skin lying anterior to the orbital septum. The first surgical step involves upper and lower lines of incisions, 1(U) and 1(L), above the superior tarsal border (STB). The second step involves an oblique transection through the orbicularis (2) via the transorbicularis vector line. For the third step (3), upon reaching and opening of the orbital septum, one dissects inferiorly towards the superior tarsal border. Step 4 shows a leveled excision of orbicularis and redundant skin above the superior tarsal border. The transorbicularis vector rotates and levels off as more skin needs to be removed, such that the cross-section of soft tissues that are debulked changes from a triangular, to a trapezoidal, and finally to a rectangular configuration. (Reproduced with permission from Chen WPD. Asian blepharoplasty: a surgical atlas. Newton: Butterworth and Heinemann; 1995: 166.)

Triangular debulking

Trapezoidal debulking

Rectangular debulking

As more tissue needs to be removed

In *triangular* debulking (without skin removal):

$$\frac{\text{Amount of Orbicularis}}{\text{Amount of Skin}} = \text{Infinity}$$

(or n, with n >> 1)

(Vertical measurement of tissues)

As you proceed to *trapezoidal* and *rectangular* debulking, the ratio of orbicularis to skin removal, as measured vertically, approaches 1:1 (with n=1).

The ratio will be below 1.0 only when the amount of skin redundancy is truly excessive, as in an elderly person, allowing the removal of excessive skin without compromising wound closure and predisposition to ectropion and lagophthalmos of the upper lid. In this situation, a 'reverse' trapezoidal block of tissue is removed, with the height over the skin side greater than the height of the preseptal orbicularis removed. Even in this case with a large amount of skin removal, the traverse through the orbicularis muscle (transorbicularis vector) should still be perpendicular to the levator palpebrae superioris muscle. Therefore:

In young individuals,

$$\frac{d\ \text{Orbicularis}}{d\ \text{Skin}} >> 1.0$$

In elderly individuals,

$$\frac{d\ \text{Orbicularis}}{d\ \text{Skin}} = 1:1,$$

and, occasionally, <1.0 (where *d* = difference)

To summarize, the applications of trapezoidal debulking of the preaponeurotic platform in Asian blepharoplasty and its advantages are as follows:

- Easier approach through the orbital septum and preaponeurotic space when the plane of dissection is beveled. It lessens the possibility of injury to the levator aponeurosis when there is a buffer of preaponeurotic fat pad under the septum and on top of the levator.

- It allows for a controlled, uniform debulking of the junctional platform of tissues in the supratarsal and pretarsal area.

- It allows optimal formation of attachments between the levator aponeurosis and the inferior subcutaneous tissues, or to the intermuscular septa within pretarsal orbicularis oculi fibers (pretarsal zone).

- It allows crease formation to be based on the individual's tarsus height.

- It reduces the rate of complications, including problems with asymmetry, shape, height, continuity, permanency, segmentation of crease caused by uneven planes of dissection, fading and late disappearance of crease, multiple creases, and persistent edema.[4]

In conclusion, this concept of triangular, trapezoidal, and rectangular debulking of the preaponeurotic platform is applicable universally to upper eyelid surgery in all ethnic groups, and in cases with challenging lid crease management problem. This latter topic will be covered in Chapter 15.

REFERENCES

1. Chen WP. Asian blepharoplasty – anatomy and technique. J Ophthalmic Plast Reconstr Surg 1987;3:135–40.
2. Collin JR, Beard C, Wood I. Experimental and clinical data on the insertion of the levator palpebrae superioris muscle. Am J Ophthalmol 1978;85:792–801.
3. Chen WP. A comparision of Caucasian and Asian blepharoplasty. Ophthalmic Pract 1991;9:216–22.
4. Chen WPD. Asian blepharoplasty: a surgical atlas. Newton, MA: Butterworth and Heinemann; 1995.
5. Chen WPD. Concept of triangular, rectangular and trapezoidal debulking of eyelid tissues: application in Asian blepharoplasty. Plast Reconstr Surg 1996;97:212–8.
6. Chen WPD. Eyelid and eyelid skin diseases. In: Lee D, Higginbotham E, eds. Clinical guide to comprehensive ophthalmology. New York: Thieme; 1998.
7. Chen WPD. Oculoplastic surgery: the essentials. New York: Thieme; 2002.
8. Sayoc BT. Plastic construction of the superior palpebral fold. Am J Ophthalmol 1954;38:556–9,1954.
9. Hayashi, K. The double eyelid operation. Jpn Rev Clin Ophthalmol 1938;33:1000–10 (Part 1);1098–110 (Part 2).
10. Fernandez LR. Double eyelid operation in the Oriental in Hawaii. Plast Reconstr Surg 1960;25:257–64.
11. Inoue, S. The double eyelid operation. Jpn Rev Clin Ophthalmol 1947;42:306.
12. Mitsui Y. Plastic construction of a double eyelid. Jpn Rev Clin Ophthalmol 1950;44:19.
13. Sayoc BT. Anatomic considerations in the plastic construction of a palpebral fold in the full upper eyelid. Am J Ophthalmol 1996;63:155–8.

Chapter 8

Lower Blepharoplasty and Primary Cheeklift

Clinton D McCord Jr

Lower Lid Blepharoplasty by Skin–muscle Flap Approach

The traditional lower blepharoplasty is indicated for patients who have aging changes, with underlying skin laxity and some gravitional descent of structures. It is also indicated for some males with aging changes who want a conservative approach.

The procedure starts by placement of a 4-0 silk as a traction suture over the central portion of the lower eyelid margin. An incisional line is marked approximately 1mm below the cilia from the medial canthus towards the lateral canthus; it is then slanted inferolaterally for approximately 6–8mm after reaching the lateral canthal angle. Ideally, the inferolateral incision would merge with one of the crow's-feet lines there (**Fig. 8.1a & b**).

The initial skin incision starts over the inferolateral portion and is best performed using a No. 15 Bard-Parker blade. Small amounts of capillary bleeding are controlled using bipolar cautery. A cutting Bovie cautery is then used to incise through the orbicularis layer to fashion a myocutaneous flap, starting at the lateral canthal area. Once a small space is initiated, a small Blair retractor is inserted and turned laterally so that the traction is lateral. Straight sharp scissors are then inserted beneath the skin over the pretarsal region, undermining the skin beneath the lashes. The incision over the infraciliary region is then completed using the straight scissors. Next, the orbicularis is undermined, and incised approximately 2–3mm below the inferior border of the tarsus, thereby avoiding the inferior tarsus arcade. The orbicularis muscle overlying the tarsus in the pretarsal region is not incised – this helps in preserving the lower lid tone. The myocutaneous flap is retracted with the Blair retractor inferiorly, while the lid margin is retracted superiorly with the traction suture or the surgeon's finger on a gauze pad.

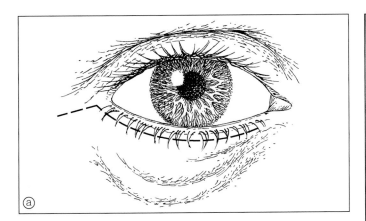

Figure 8.1 (a) Infraciliary incision line for lower blepharoplasty.

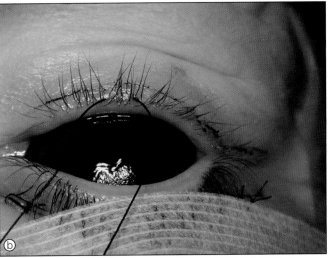

Figure 8.1 (b) Upside down view of right lower eyelid (surgeon's view).

Gentle pressure on the globe allows any fat to protrude forward. A Bovie needle is then used to incise the septum (**Fig. 8.2**). Incision into the central fat pocket is done first. Prolapsing and redundant fat may be excised using a combination of bipolar cautery first, followed by excision using the Bovie needle on coagulation mode. The retractor is then repositioned towards the nasal direction, retracting the medial edge of the lower lid incision nasally, and with downward pressure the nasal fat pad is made to protrude. The capsule is incised and the nasal fat pad, which is usually pale white, may protrude. The fat is similarly excised using bipolar cautery as well as the Bovie needle on coagulation mode. Any visible blood vessels should be carefully cauterized before allowing them to be reposited. Between the central and nasal fat pads lies the inferior oblique muscle and this should be protected. The lateral fat pocket is removed, if necessary, after the lateral canthoplasty procedure is performed.

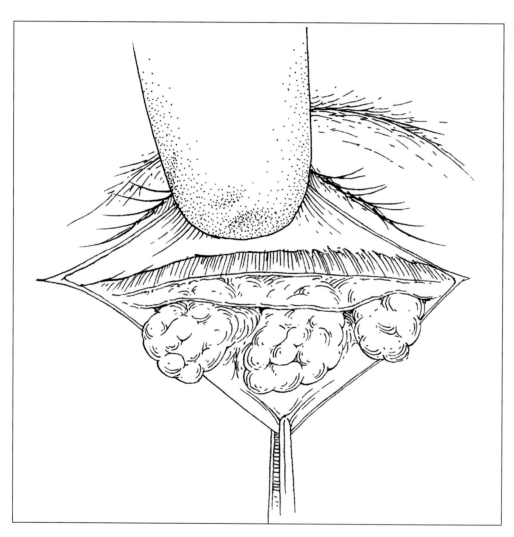

Figure 8.2

Surgical technique of lateral canthoplasty

Often a patient will exhibit age-related laxity of the lower lid margin as well as lateral canthal dehiscence. The addition of this maneuver allows the surgeon to stabilize the eyelid fissure, correct for horizontal laxity of the lower eyelid, as well as adjust for the prominent-eye patient as seen in thyroid eye disease. This is performed before the lateral fat pad excision because it will affect the prominence of the lateral fat pad.

A lateral canthotomy is performed using scissors, connecting the incision with the inferolateral extension of the skin incision line. An inferior cantholysis is performed over the superficial and deep portion of the lateral canthal tendon. The freed lower lid segment is draped under mild tension against the globe and directed towards a point just above the lateral orbital tubercle in the area of the lateral orbital rim. A redundant segment of the lower lid, measuring between 2 and 5mm, may be excised, depending on individual findings. Capillary oozing from the inferior tarsal aracade is easily stopped with bipolar cautery. The reanchoring of the lateral portion of the tarsus may be performed using either a 5-0 Vicryl or 4-0 Prolene suture on a P-2 needle (Ethicon) (**Fig. 8.3**). The needle is inserted through the inferior portion of the tarsus, taking an intratarsal bite and then exiting through the upper portion of the tarsal plate, just below the lid margin so that it will remain buried when tied. This upper end of the suture is then passed through the inner periorbita just above the lateral orbital tubercle and brought from inside the lateral orbital rim outward. It is then reinserted from outside the lateral orbital rim inward and tightened with a double throw until the lower lid margin rests along the lower corneal limbus with the desired tension. Lid tension is tested intraoperatively to confirm appropriate tightness. In persons who do not show any laxity and in whom no excision of the lateral portion of the lower lid is performed, the tied suture may even contain slack. When the knots are tied, care is taken to make sure that the suture knot will not protrude and irritate the overlying skin.

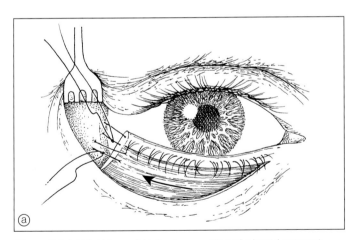

Figure 8.3 (a) Right lower lid following resection of a lateral segment.

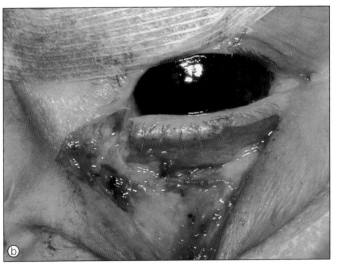

Figure 8.3 (b) Right lower lid following resection of a lateral segment.

Undermining of the skin–muscle flap

It is important to undermine the skin–muscle flap over the malar area separating the septal strands and periosteum from the myocutaneous flap (**Fig. 8.4a & b**). This allows for further smoothing of the malar area. Failure to do this will cause anterior distortion of the lateral fat pocket, requiring more resection. Once the myocutaneous flap is dissected free, the lateral fat pocket may be resected if necessary.

Lateral fat pad excision

The lateral fat pad may be trimmed with a combination of bipolar and Bovie cautery following horizontal tightening and undermining of the skin–muscle flap. It is important to preserve the arcuate portion of the orbital septum laterally, to prevent recurrence of the lateral fat pad prolapse. The lateral fat and the central fat are connected and can be teased from behind this portion of the septum without severing it.

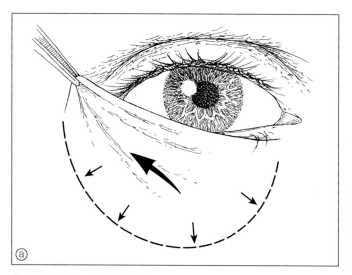
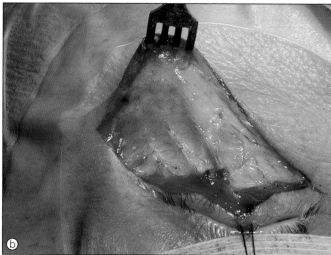

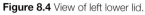
Figure 8.4 View of left lower lid.

Resection of the skin–muscle flap and periosteal fixation

The tip of the skin–muscle flap is stretched towards the superior tip of the ear to determine how much the lateral portion of the flap overlaps the underlying incision (**Fig. 8.5a**). The first triangle of excess tissue is excised from the lateral portion of the skin–muscle flap. The flap is sutured at the lateral canthal angle's lateral periosteum to create a desired level of tension over the cheekbone and correct for any hollowing effect in the lower lid. Trial positioning of the flap to the lateral rim may be performed until the desired level of tension is obtained. For this maneuver, a 4-0 silk suture is used: it passes through the anchoring point located on the skin–muscle flap, then into the lateral periosteum at the desired position, and is then brought out through the skin–muscle layer of the upper edge of the lower blepharoplasty incision at the lateral canthal area (**Figs. 8.5b & 8.6**). The second triangle of excess skin–muscle flap is then trimmed along the infraciliary incision line. This is usually a long and thin triangular strip.

Trimming of the orbicularis muscle fibers from beneath the skin–muscle flap may be performed if there seems to be excess, to further thin the lid down. These are orbicularis fibers that overlap the muscle fibers deliberately left on the pretarsal area from the original incision. This is more applicable to women, to give a smooth look; in men, it is often left in place, to avoid an overly thinned appearance. The flap is everted and examined for bleeders; any vessels that are actively bleeding are cauterized with bipolar cautery.

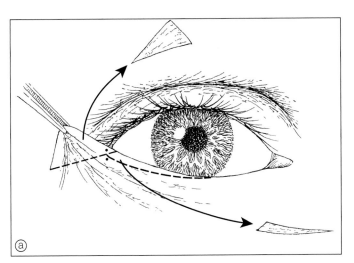

Figure 8.5 (a) Segment of redundancy removed in lower blepharoplasty.

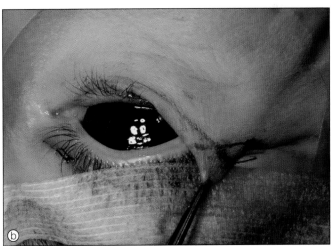

Figure 8.5 (b) Right lower lid.

Figure 8.6 Upside down view of right lower lid.

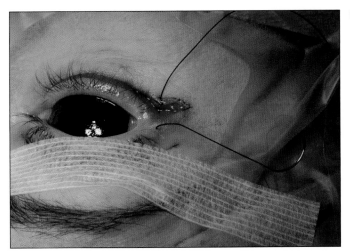

Wound closure

Closure of the skin flap is performed using 7-0 silk sutures. The inferolateral region of the incision is best closed using a vertical mattress suture, taking care that both the skin edge and the deeper orbicularis are closed. The vertical mattress suture is placed with alternating deep bites through skin and orbicularis and shallower bites through skin and subcutaneous tissues. An alternative to this is the utilization of a 'far-near-near-far' type of baseball stitching using 7-0 silk, which gives good wound approximation as well as tension control (**Fig. 8.7a & b**). Meticulous closure is essential in this conspicuous area in order to avoid scarring. A small dog-ear may be seen laterally and can be trimmed off.

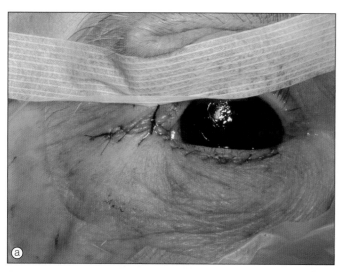

Figure 8.7 (a) Closure of blepharoplasty wound in right lower lid.

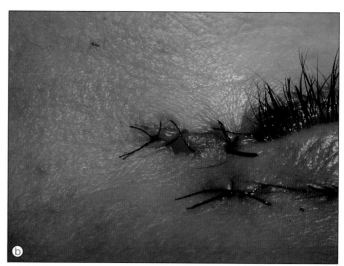

Figure 8.7 (b) Closure of blepharoplasty wound in left lower lid.

The Primary Cheeklift

The traditional lower blepharoplasty has only limited value in addressing anyone with significant gravitational ptosis of the midface or cheek, which is present in the majority of middle-aged patients. The lower eyelid should not be considered as a structure that ages in isolation and behaves independently of the supporting contiguous structures beneath it. It is therefore best evaluated as part of the midface structure which is subjected to the same involutional laxity, ligamentous dehiscences, and atrophy, as well as gravitational sagging. Lower blepharoplasty can therefore be performed as part of the midface rejuvenation made possible through a cheeklift.

The cheeklift addresses the aging changes that occur in the triangular area from the nasolabial fold to the eyelids:

- eyelid fat protrusion;

- laxity and sagging of eyelid skin and midface skin; and

- descent of subcutaneous face fat and midface structures.

Subcutaneous sagging of orbicularis muscle and dropping of the malar fat pad cause a good part of the changes that occur with age – when they are repositioned, this restores the face to a more youthful appearance (see Fig. 2.14).

The trans-lid cheeklift (**Fig. 8.8a**) repositions the cheek in a more anatomically correct vector than the facelift. The traditional facelift (**Fig. 8.8b**) should be more properly called a necklift with oblique vectors towards the ear – the vertical-upward vector is the proper direction to restore the cheek and midface contours.

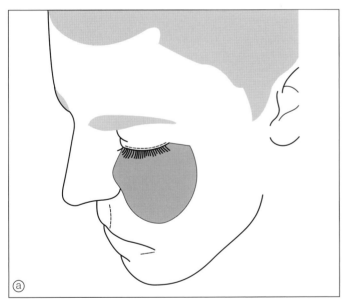

Figure 8.8 (a) Trans-lid cheeklift

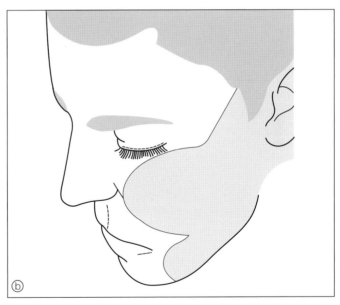

Figure 8.8 (b) Traditional facelift.

With our development of the trans-lid cheeklift, we now limit the dissection for facelift towards the neck area (**Fig. 8.8c**), while the midface area is addressed exclusively through the lower lid.

To briefly review the anatomic layers of the midface (see Figs 2.15–2.21):

■ The first layer, facial bone, shows the sensory nerves and origin of some facial mimetic muscles.

■ The next layer shows the mimetic muscles in place – the levator labii insertions at the orbital rim nasally are included in the dissection.

■ Then, on top of the mimetic muscles and under the orbicularis muscle, is a layer of fat called the sub-orbicularis oculi fat (SOOF), which extends to the brow to become the retro-orbicularis oculi fat (ROOF).

■ The next layer is the orbicularis muscle.

■ A deep portion of the malar fat pad lies on top of the orbicularis and is just under and permeated by the superficial musculo-aponeurotic system (SMAS).

■ The SMAS overlies the previous deep portion of the malar fat – and in turn the superficial portion of the malar fat lies above it. The SMAS is blocked inferiorly by the nasolabial fold.

■ And on top of that is the skin.

One other structure that is important, which originates from the orbital rim and combines with (and is considered to be part of) the SMAS, is the orbital malar ligament.

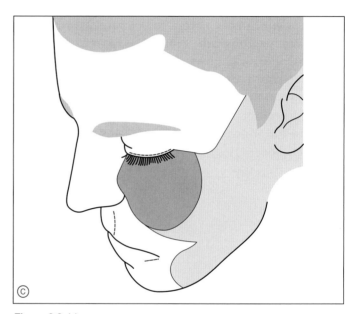

Figure 8.8 (c)

Surgical steps of the cheeklift

The cheeklift mechanics should be thought of as composing of two important steps:

- anchoring of the canthus, which mainly controls the shape of the eyelid fissure; and

- anchoring of the cheek flap itself (inferior orbicularis arc), which really supports the lower lid and cheek

The skin–muscle flap is elevated and dissected to the inferior rim where the periosteum is incised. **Figure 8.9** shows the subperiosteal dissection of the flap from the rim, elevating the cheek tissue from the cheekbone.

The subperiosteal elevation is carried out over the zygomatic area but stops short of the nerve nasally – the periosteum usually needs release, particularly over the zygomatic area (**Fig. 8.10**).

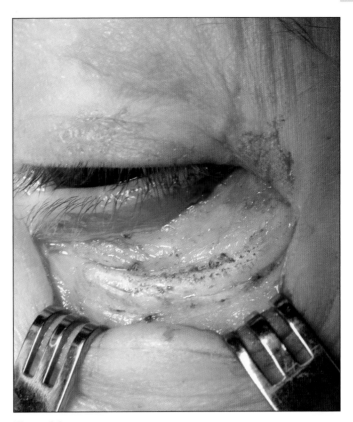

Figure 8.9

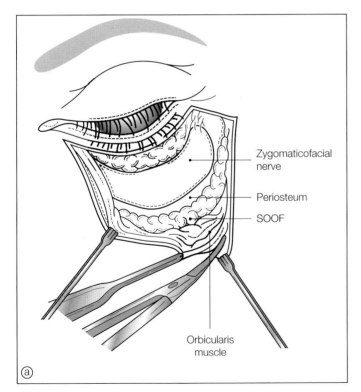

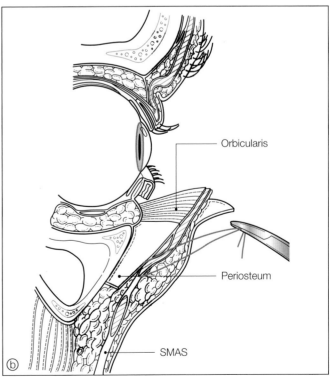

Figure 8.10

Further release is obtained by finger stretching (**Fig. 8.11**).

The first of the two anchoring procedures is at the lateral canthus. Anchoring at the canthus controls the shape of the eyelid fissure. In patients with standard eye prominence, unmodified canthal anchoring can be used (**Fig. 8.12**). The canthus is anchored at the level of inferior pupil edge and inside the lateral orbital rim. It is important always to include the upper lid in the fixation, for alignment and function of eyelid closure.

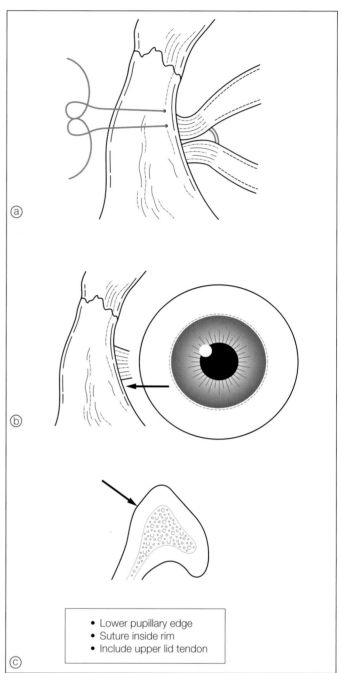

- Lower pupillary edge
- Suture inside rim
- Include upper lid tendon

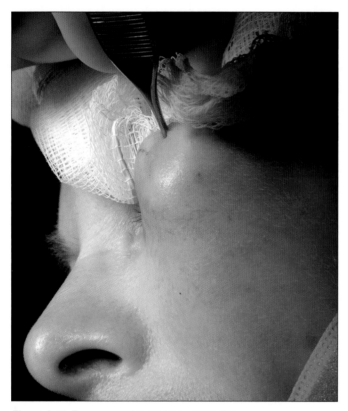

Figure 8.11 Finger stretching to loosen cheek flap.

Figure 8.12 Canthal anchoring – standard eye prominence.

With a deep-set or enophthalmic eye, and the prominent (or proptotic) eye, the horizontal direction of pull must be modified to prevent the clotheslining upward in the deep-set eye, or, conversely, the clotheslining downward in the prominent eye (**Fig. 8.13**).

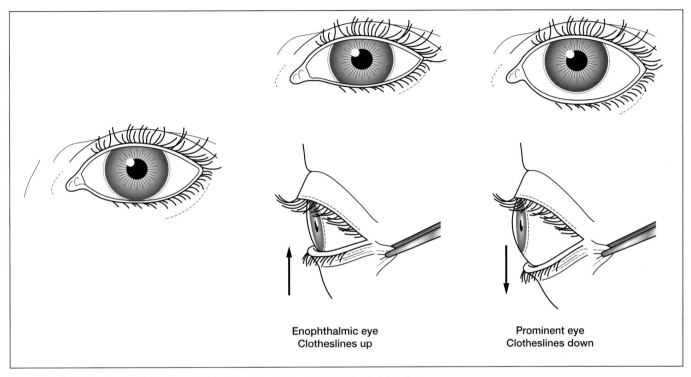

Enophthalmic eye
Clotheslines up

Prominent eye
Clotheslines down

Figure 8.13 Effect of horizontal vector with lateral canthoplasty orbicularis–cheek tightening.

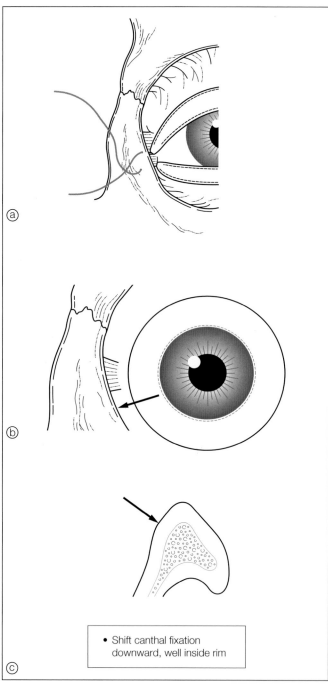

Figure 8.14 Canthoplasty – enophthalmic eye.

Upward clotheslining in the deep-set eye produces an overly narrow fissure – a 'squinty' eye. Thus, with the deep-set eye, canthal anchoring is shifted downward and more internal, to prevent such effect (**Figs 8.14 & 8.15**).

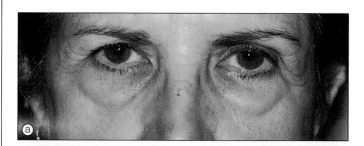

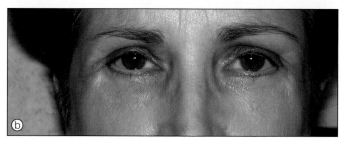

Figure 8.15 A patient with a deep-set eye – Hertel 15 – before and after a cheeklift with modification of canthal anchoring.

Downward clotheslining in the prominent eye produces scleral show. Thus, with a prominent eye, canthal anchoring is shifted upward, usually with slack, to prevent such effect (**Figs 8.16 & 8.17**).

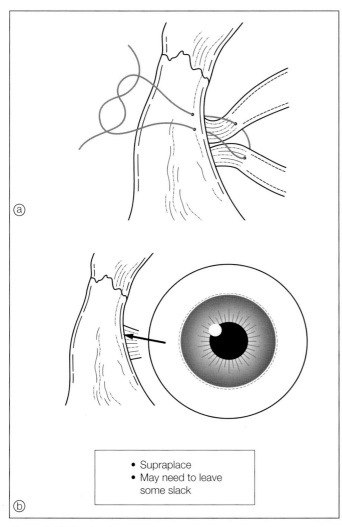

Figure 8.16 Canthoplasty – prominent eye.

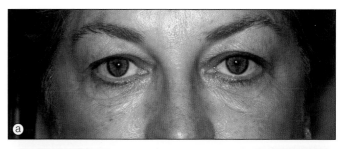
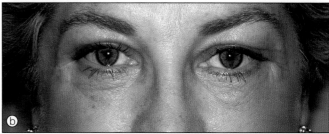

Figure 8.17 A patient with prominent eyes – Hertel 18+ – a little over a week after a canthoplasty modified for the prominent eye.

With lower lid laxity (redundancy), tightening of the tarsoligamentous sling prevents buckling of the lower lid and ectropion (**Fig. 8.18**).

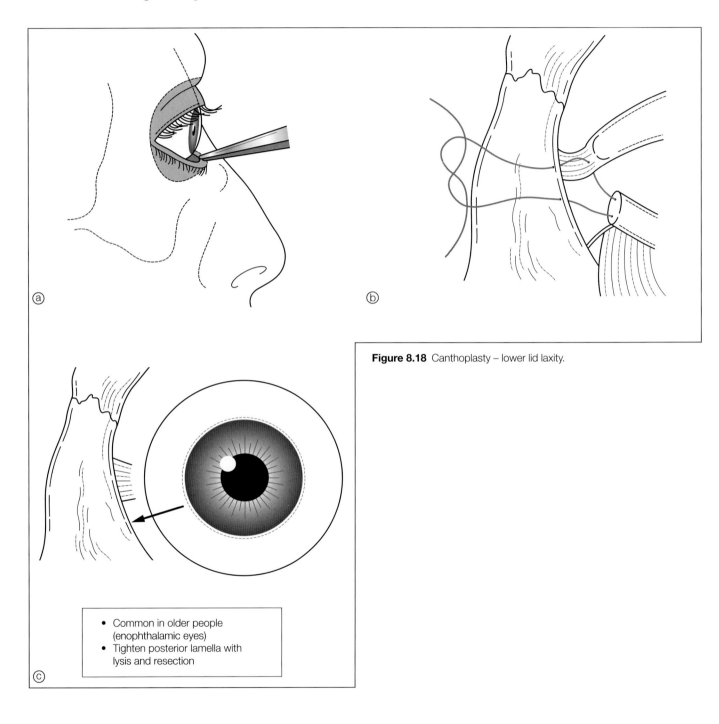

Figure 8.18 Canthoplasty – lower lid laxity.

- Common in older people (enophthalamic eyes)
- Tighten posterior lamella with lysis and resection

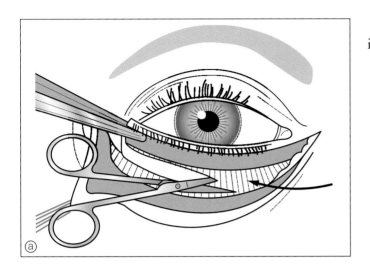

With increasing prominence, I routinely release the inferior retractors (capsulo-palpebral fascia) (**Fig. 8.19**).

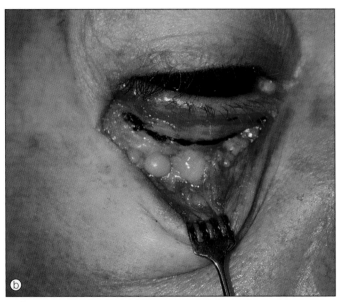

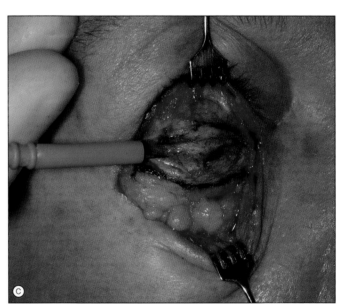

Figure 8.19 Recession of capsulo-palpebral fascia.

With cases of more severe prominence, use of a primary spacer prevents postoperative scleral show – right now, Alloderm seems to work well (**Figs 8.20 & 8.21**).

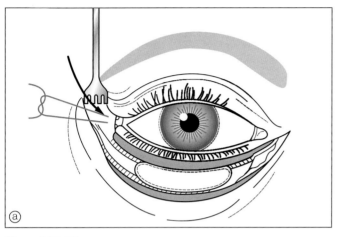

Figure 8.20 Primary spacer.

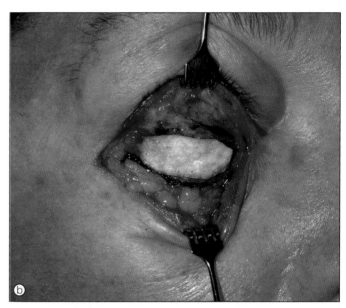

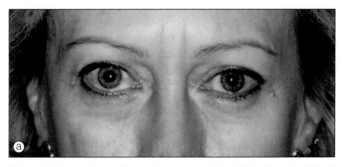

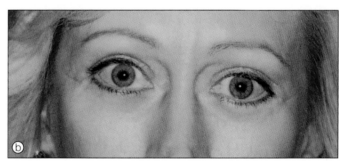

Figure 8.21 A patient with prominent eyes – Hertel 19 – after cheeklift with primary spacer.

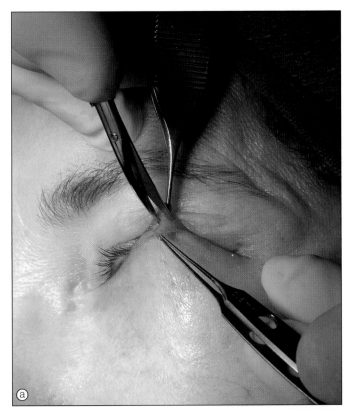

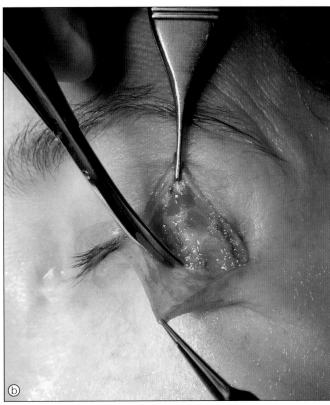

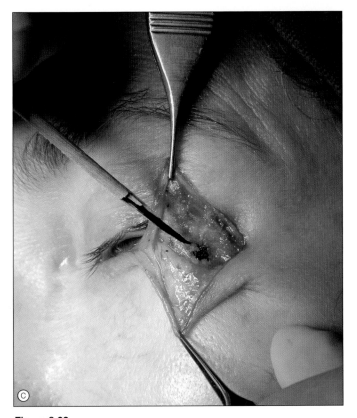

The other major anchoring step is anchoring the inferior arc of the orbicularis muscle in the cheeklift flap. This supports the lower lid and the cheek.

To isolate a portion of the inferior arc of the orbicularis muscle, a subcutaneous dissection is performed down to the inferior edge of the muscle into the SMAS (**Fig. 8.22**).

Figure 8.22

The muscle flap usually will be pulled in a different vector than the skin flap (**Fig. 8.23**).

The anchoring of the orbicularis muscle is very important – it is the *handle of the cheeklift.* With its fixation and anchoring, it *redrapes the cheek* and it also *provides a sling-like support for the lower lid.* Also, with its redraping, the *eyelid fat is repositioned* by tension of the flap on the orbital septum which lines the inner surface of the flap.

Double anchoring is necessary – the *base* of the orbicularis muscle arc is anchored at the orbital rim at the level of the lateral canthus, while the *tip* of the orbicularis muscle arc is anchored at varying places in the deep temporal fascia (**Fig. 8.24**).

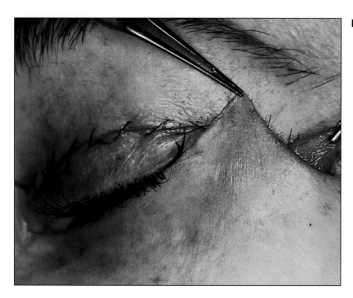

Figure 8.23 Development of orbicularis flap.

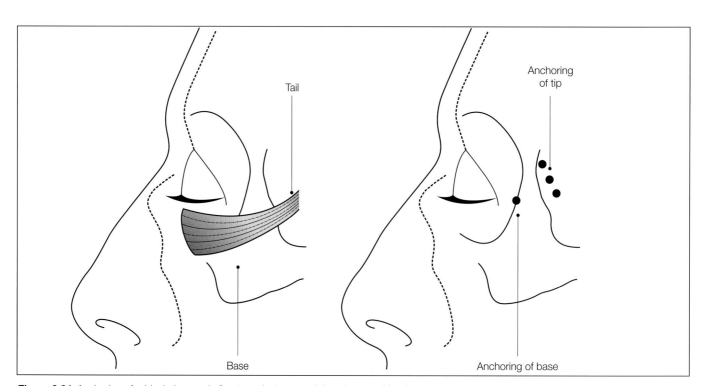

Figure 8.24 Anchoring of orbicularis muscle flap to periosteum and deep temporal fascia.

Before fixation of the muscle occurs, there are variations in the redraping of the orbicularis muscle flap.

In the non-prominent eye, an oblique or more horizontal vector can be used for attachment of the base of the flap for optimal smoothing of the cheek and the nasolabial fold (**Fig. 8.25**).

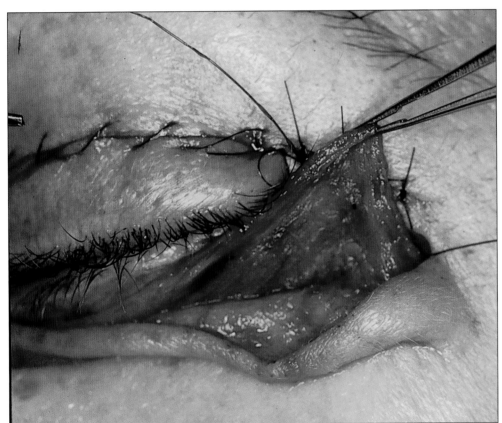

Figure 8.25 Non-prominent eye.

In patients with a prominent eye, a vertical vector must be used to prevent the clotheslining effect on the lower lid (**Fig. 8.26**).

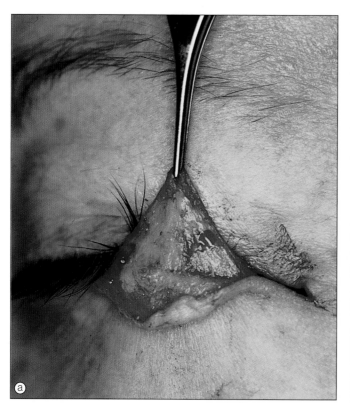 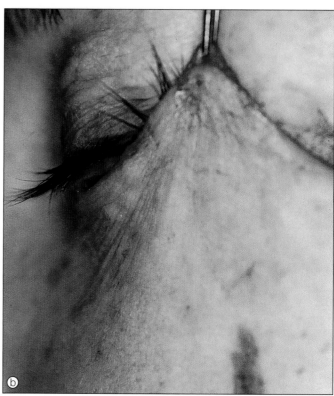

Figure 8.26 Prominent eye.

The fixating suture for anchoring the base of the flap is placed at the inferior edge of the orbicularis – in the SMAS (**Fig. 8.27a**).

Before the suture is placed in the flap, the anchoring suture is first double-looped stitched in the periosteum at the lateral orbital rim (**Fig. 8.27b**).

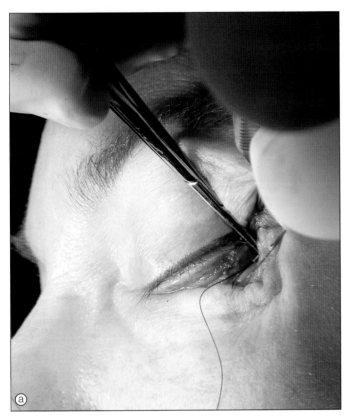 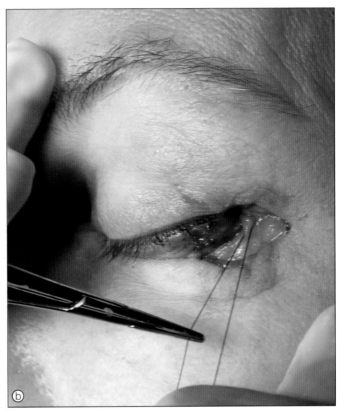

Figure 8.27 Periosteal stitch.

It is then brought through the muscle–SMAS flap with a quilting suture (**Fig. 8.28a,b**).

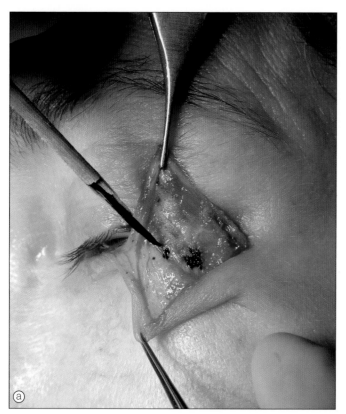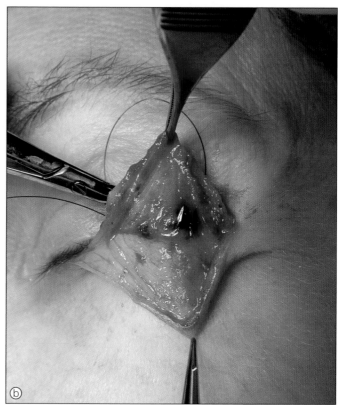

Figure 8.28

After anchoring the base of the flap at the orbital rim, the tip of the flap is then fixated to the deep temporal fascia (**Fig. 8.29a,b**).

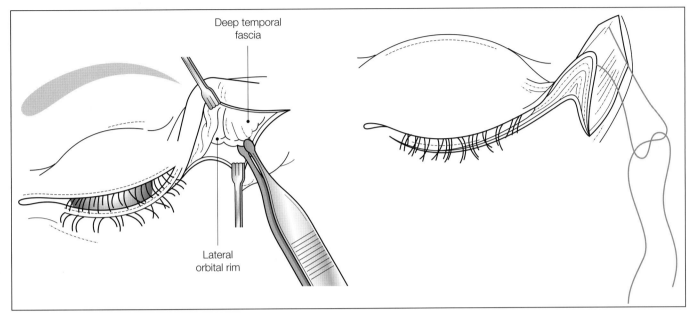

Figure 8.29 Fixation of tip of flap.

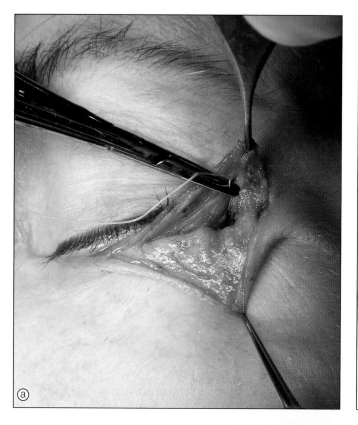

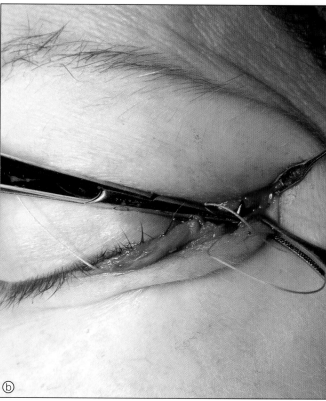

Figure 8.30 shows suturing the tip of the flap to the deep temporal fascia – some redundant muscle is usually trimmed.

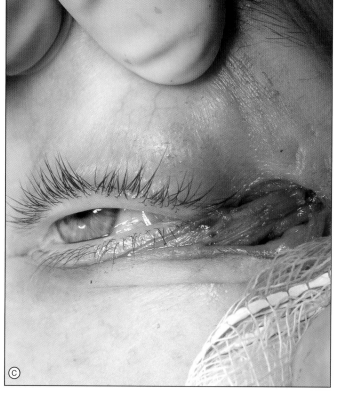

Figure 8.30

A good bit of skin is usually vertically recruited over the lateral half of the lid margin; it may be excised after careful assessment (**Fig. 8.31a & b**).

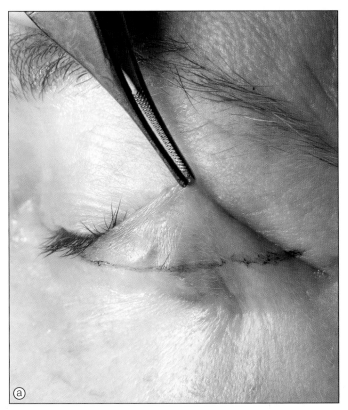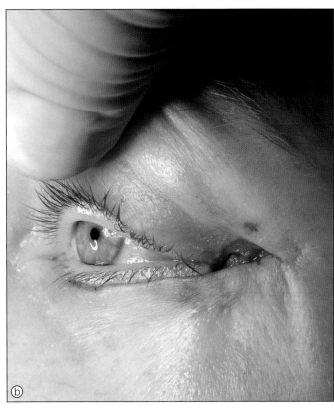

Figure 8.31

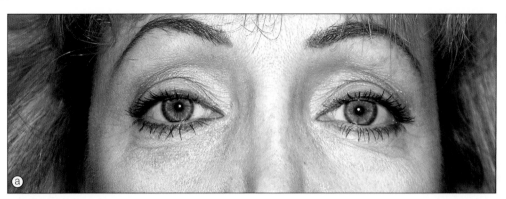

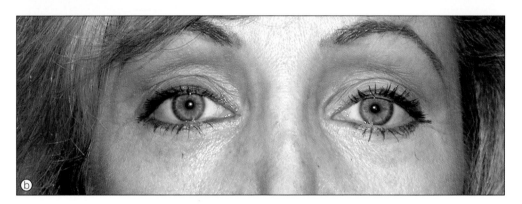

Figure 8.32 (a) Before and (b) after.

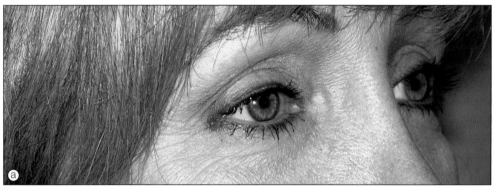

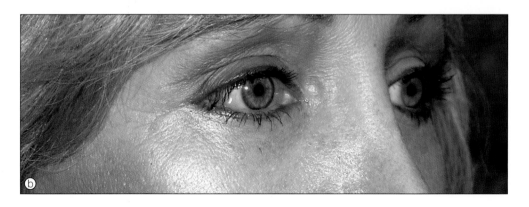

Figure 8.33 Oblique views. (a) Before and (b) after.

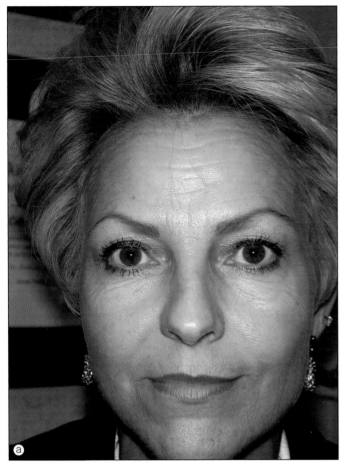
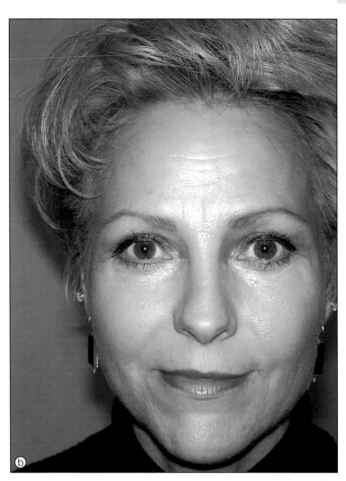

Figure 8.34 (a) Before and (b) after.

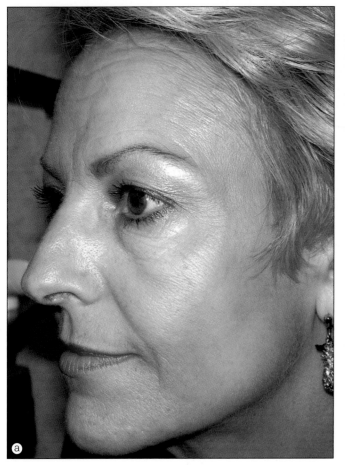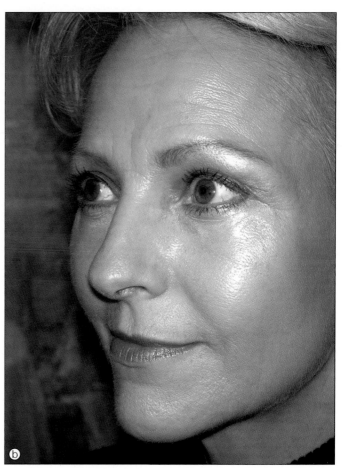

Figure 8.35 (a) Before and (b) after.

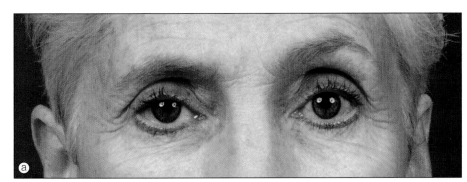

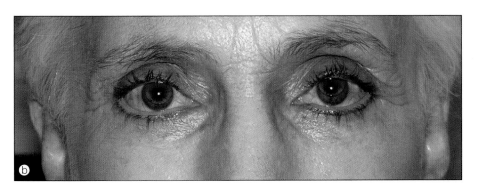

Figure 8.36 Frontal view. (a) Before and (b) after.

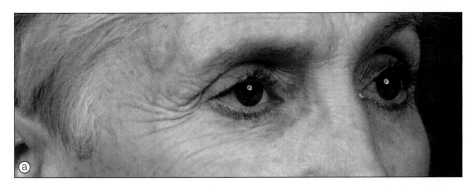

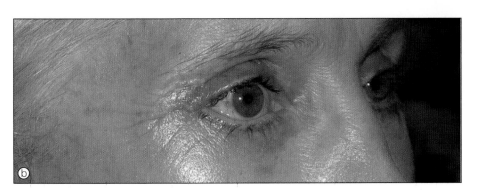

Figure 8.37 Oblique view. (a) Before and (b) after.

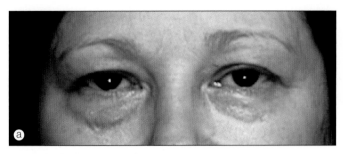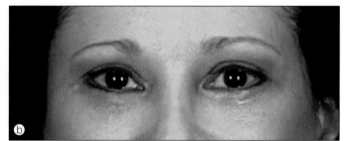

Figure 8.38 (a) Before and (b) after.

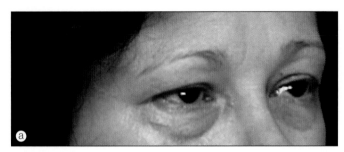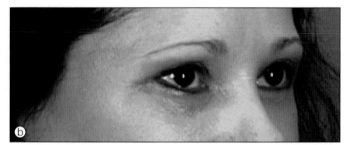

Figure 8.39 (a) Before and (b) after.

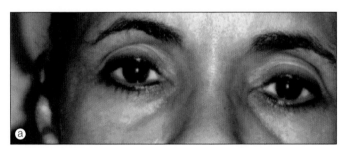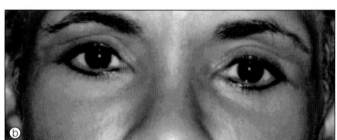

Figure 8.40 (a) Before and (b) after.

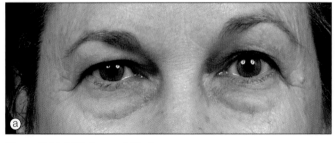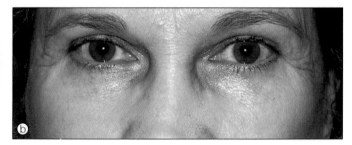

Figure 8.41 (a) Before and (b) after.

Recently, I reviewed 195 cheeklift procedures performed over approximately 18 months, 151 of which were primary cheeklifts. Using the described techniques, only four cases (2.6%) required any revision – a rate that is quite acceptable for a cosmetic procedure.

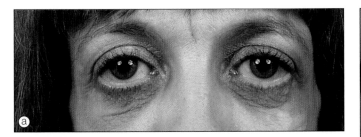

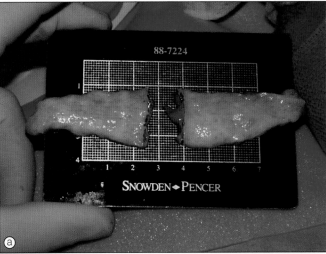

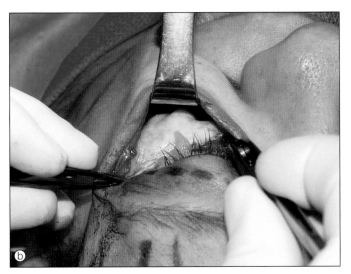

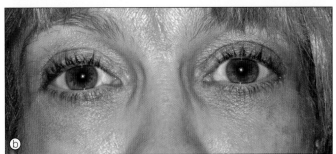

Figure 8.42 A special case – a patient with facial dystrophy and severe eye prominence. Dermis fat grafts were placed in the malar area as a cheek filler. Dr Foad Nahai worked on the lower face of this patient.

Figure 8.43 I was responsible for the eyelids and cheek and used a primary spacer of autogenous dermis to normalize the eyelid fissure.

Avoidance of Complications with Lower Lid Blepharoplasty Cheeklift

Clinton D McCord Jr

Chapter 9

Anchoring techniques are the heart of not only the prevention of problems but also the correction of problems.

The term 'anchoring' refers to the two main fixation points in a cheeklift:

- *anchoring of the lateral eyelid tendons –* canthoplasty or pexy, which controls the *shape* of the *eyelid fissure*; and

- *anchoring of the inferior arch of the orbicularis muscle*, which provides *support* for the lower lid and *positions the mid-cheek*.

The approach to the lower lid surgery is to perform cheeklifts through transcutaneous eyelid incisions with optimum redraping of skin.

The two most common problems after cheeklift are:

- abnormalities in the shape of the eyelid fissure from failure of *canthal anchoring*; and

- retraction and sagging of the lower lid and cheek from failure of anchoring of the *inferior orbicularis muscle*.

Eyelid fissure shape is the result of the position and curvature of the upper and lower lids. Excellent studies have shown mathematically that upper lid curvature is almost solely the result of the indentation of the globe on the lid. This is not so with the lower lid, where indentation does play some role, but the tone and position and laxity of the canthal attachments of the lower lid are the most important.

Normal eyelid fissure shape varies, but, in general, the lower lid edge reaches the inferior limbus – the canthal angle is as high as the inferior pupillary edge.

The downward displacement of the canthus and lower lid that occurs with age is a constant.

Figure 9.1 summarizes the variety of modifications that must be made in lateral canthoplasties with the varying conditions of:

- a standard positioned eye;
- a lower lid with horizontal laxity;
- a prominent eye; and
- an enophthalmic eye.

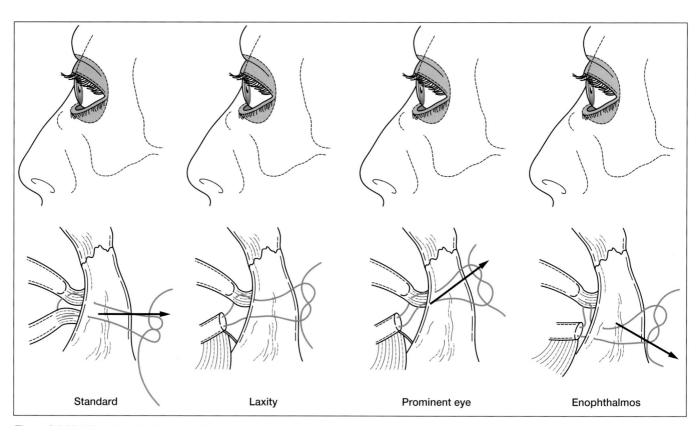

| Standard | Laxity | Prominent eye | Enophthalmos |

Figure 9.1 Variations in canthal anchoring (lateral canthoplasty) technique.

Patients with a greater degree of eye prominence usually will require additional steps to prevent scleral show. *Loosening of the retractors in the lower lid by recession of the capsulo-palpebral fascia will gain some upward movement of the lid edge in prominent-eyed patients* (see Fig. 8.19). Those with very prominent eyes will require primary insertion of spacer material (see Fig. 8.20). This may include autogenous fascia lata or autologous dermis (Alloderm) primarily to elevate the lower lid margin to prevent scleral show.

It is the anchoring of the flap of the inferior arc of the orbicularis muscle that is the handle of the cheek-lift and acts as a sling to support the lower lid.

The suborbicularis oculi fat (SOOF) and malar fat are fused to the muscle by the interdigitation of the superficial musculo-aponeurotic system (SMAS) and are redraped upward as the muscle is redraped.

Periorbital eyelid fat and prolapsed anterior orbital fat are repositioned by the tension of the reanchored flap on the orbital septum, which is on the posterior surface of the muscle flap.

Double anchoring of the orbicularis muscle flap is necessary: the base of the muscle flap is anchored in the periosteum at the lateral rim, while the tip of the muscle flap is anchored at varying places in the deep temporal fascia superolateral to the lateral orbital tubercle (see Fig. 8.24).

The vector of redraping of the muscle flap must vary according to eye prominence. In the non-prominent eye, a more oblique vector can be used for maximum smoothing. With prominent eyes, a vertical vector of redraping must be used to prevent the downward clotheslining effect.

There are many techniques described to perform the cheeklift from a distant incision, with different vectors needed for canthal anchoring and muscle flap anchoring. However, because of the variations in eye prominence and laxity, it is difficult to see how performing a cheeklift from a single remote vector can take into account these needed variations.

Figure 9.2

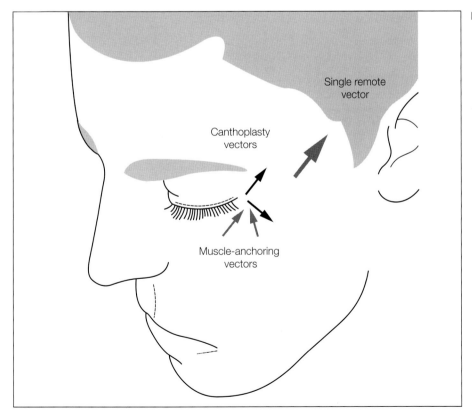

In many patients, there may be combined reasons for problems. When selecting a procedure to correct a problem following cheeklift, it is important to choose one that is anatomically appropriate.

The complications that occur following cheeklifts need to be accurately diagnosed as:

- primarily an *anchoring* problem;

- primarily a skin *shortage* problem; or

- failure to recognize *eye prominence*.

To summarize the techniques needed to correct postoperative problems following cheeklifts:

- anchoring – muscle flap, canthus – through lateral canthoplasty, orbicularis muscle flap, periosteal flap;

- skin recruitment – vertical skin recruitment with a secondary cheeklift, by reanchoring the orbicularis flap; and

- use of spacer – for prominent eyes and in scarring.

With regards to problems arising from poor anchoring at the canthus (canthal anchoring for fissure abnormalities), three reconstructive procedures are available:

- a repeat simple canthoplasty, for simple shape problems;

- periosteal flap canthoplasty (**Fig. 9.3a**); and

- canthoplasty with fascia sling to the lower lid (**Fig. 9.3b**).

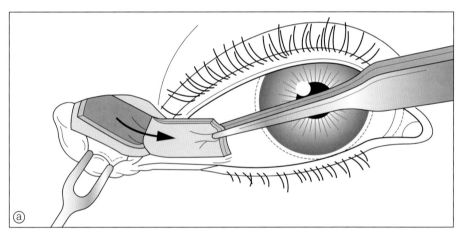

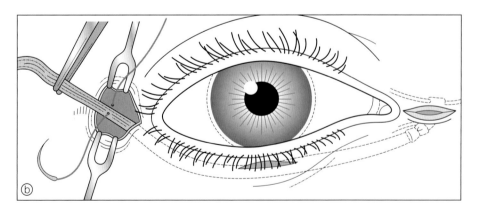

Figure 9.3 Reconstructive anchoring procedures for the lateral canthus. (a) Periosteal strip canthoplasty. (b) Fascia sling canthoplasty.

If stronger anchoring is needed:

- Phimosis and too much upward slant is corrected by reanchoring with a simple canthoplasty at 1 week (**Fig. 9.4**).

- Too much downward slant is corrected by reanchoring with a simple canthoplasty (**Fig. 9.5**).

Figure 9.4

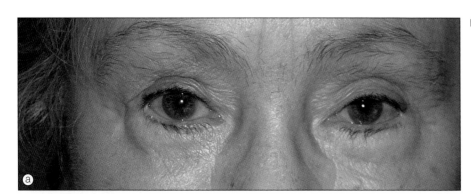

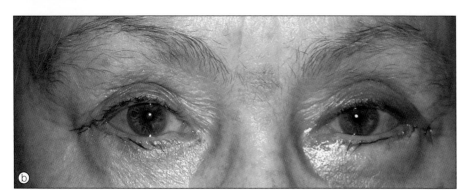

Figure 9.5

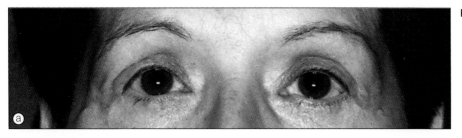

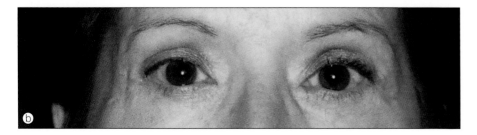

Good canthal anchoring is needed for eyelid closure. Normally, there is a very firm attachment of the tarsal plates at the lateral rim, so that when the circular orbicularis muscles contract, the circular contracture is translated into a vertical vector, resulting in apposition of the lid margins (upper lid coming down and lower lid going up). With good anchoring laterally, a vertical vector of closure is restored by the firm canthal anchoring. With poor anchoring, the vertical vector of closure is lost, so that when the circular muscles contract, it creates fishmouthing with poor closure of the eyelids.

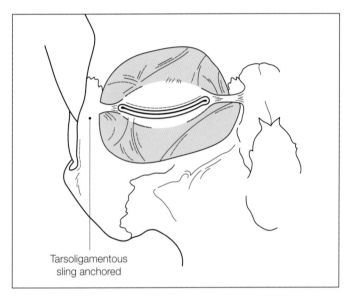

Tarsoligamentous sling anchored

Figure 9.6

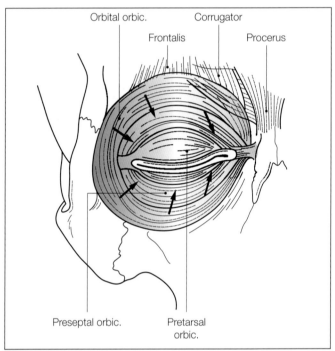

Figure 9.7

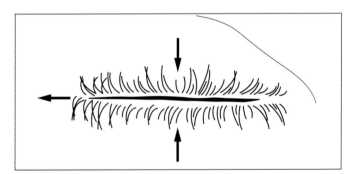

Figure 9.8 Normal blinking and closure of eyelids.

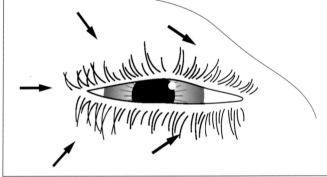

Figure 9.9 Poor closure – fishmouthing seen in poor canthal position or anchoring.

These closure problems can be subtle. For example, there was a patient with chronic chemosis. Several plastic surgeons and an experienced oculoplastic surgeon referred her for evaluation. Her chemosis was refractory to all medical treatment (**Figs 9.10 & 9.11**).

On close inspection, I noticed a mild fishmouthing and poor closure. She did have corneal signs of mild exposure. One week after canthal anchoring and cheeklift revision, good eyelid closure and complete clearing of the chemosis were achieved (**Fig. 9.12**).

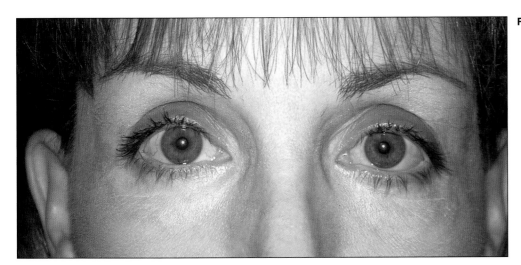

Figure 9.10

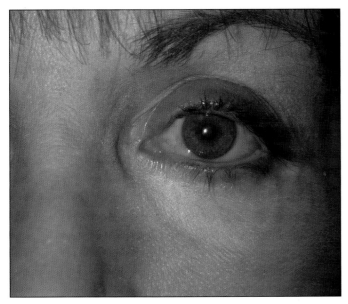

Figure 9.11

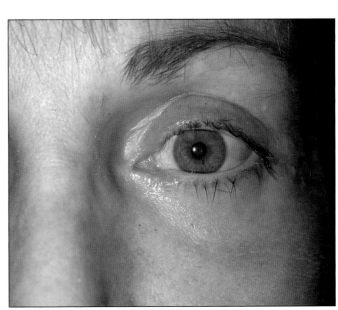

Figure 9.12

The patient shown in **Figure 9.13** exhibited postoperative phimosis or narrowing of the fissure, which was resistant to simple canthoplasty. This was corrected by reanchoring with a periosteal strip canthoplasty.

Figures **9.14 & 9.15** similarly show correction by canthoplasty and fascia sling.

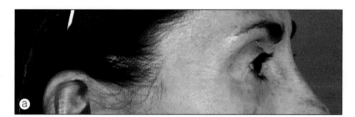
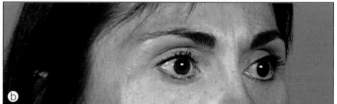

Figure 9.13

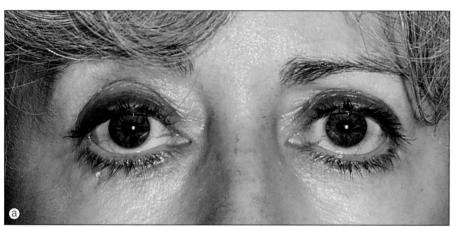

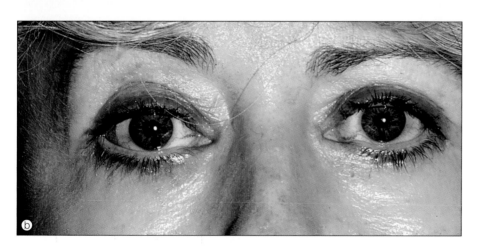

Figure 9.14 Canthoplasty with fascia sling. (a) Before and (b) after.

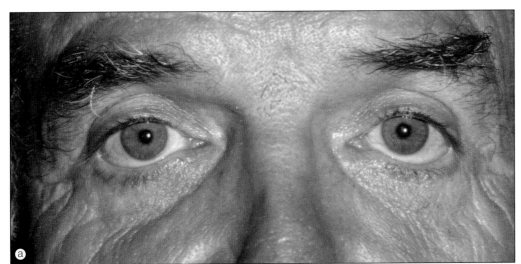

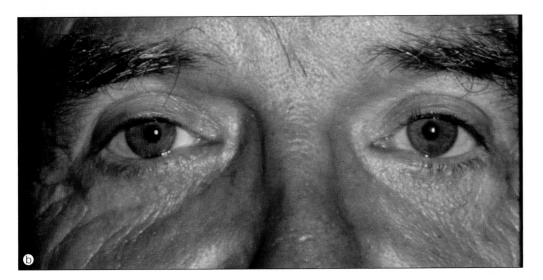

Figure 9.15 Canthoplasty with fascia sling. (a) Before and (b) after.

The other major anchoring problem can occur in the muscle flap supporting the cheek and lid – slippage can result in a relative shortage of skin. In patients with severe skin deficiency, a *secondary* cheeklift with vertical reanchoring of the muscle flap will produce an amazing amount of vertical recruitment of skin into the lower lid (**Figs 9.16–9.22**).

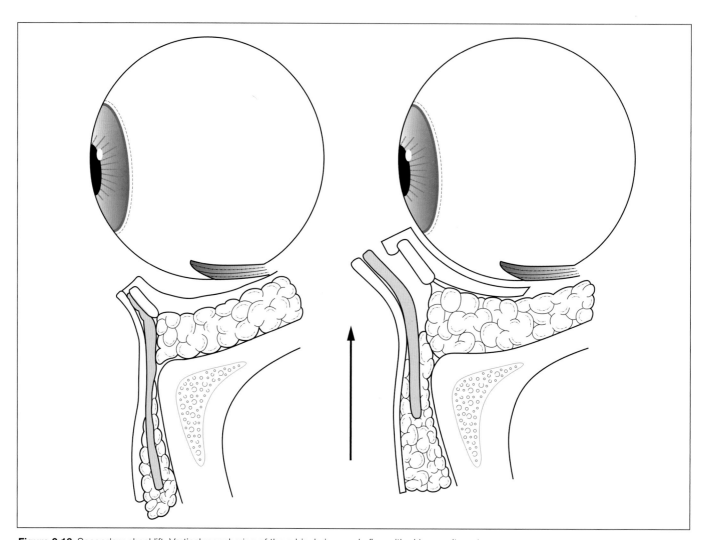

Figure 9.16 Secondary cheeklift. Vertical reanchoring of the orbicularis muscle flap with skin recruitment

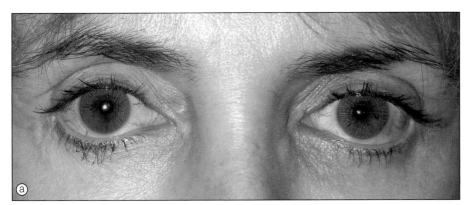

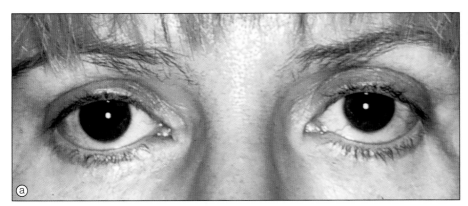

Figure 9.17 Skin-deficient lids – correction by secondary cheeklift.

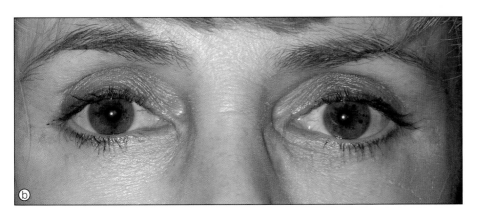

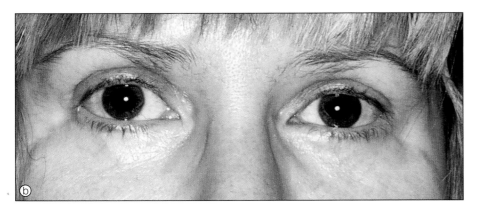

Figure 9.18 Skin-deficient lids – correction by secondary cheeklift.

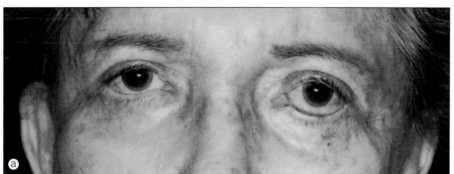

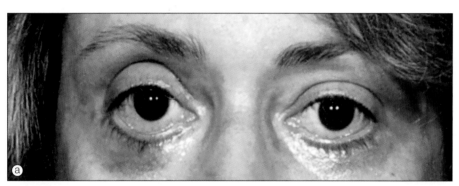

Figure 9.19 Skin-deficient lids – correction by secondary cheeklift.

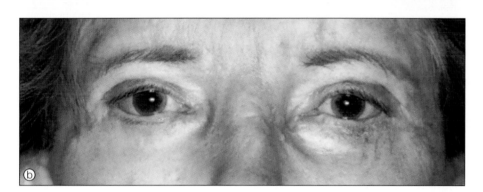

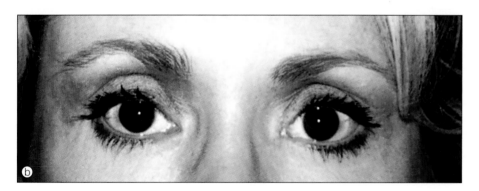

Figure 9.20 A more challenging case for skin recruitment. Correction by secondary cheeklift. Reanchoring and recruitment twice was needed.

Dr Rod Hester of Atlanta and I used staged excision of scars and skin recruitment with secondary anchoring procedures. I was responsible for the eyelids with anchoring procedures. We were able to get to this point. She has only recently had very small skin grafts at the outside corner of the lids (**Fig. 9.22**).

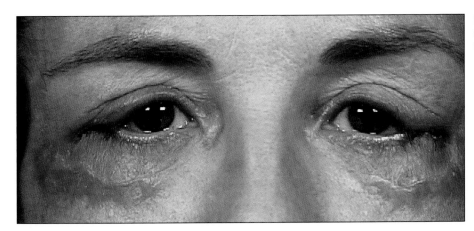

Figure 9.21 This was the greatest challenge to date for skin recruitment – laser burns from resurfacing.

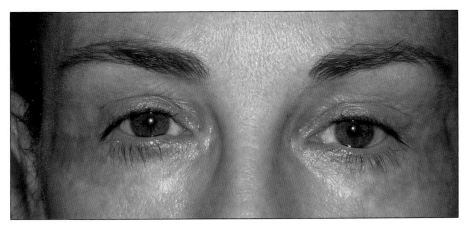

Figure 9.22 Same patient as in Figure 9.21, showing very small skin grafts at the outside corner of the lids.

The situation may arise when the periosteum is inadequate for reanchoring of the muscle flap (**Fig. 9.23A**) – if so, a drill hole is needed for anchoring.

This is most commonly placed at the lateral canthus (**Figs 9.23B & 9.24**).

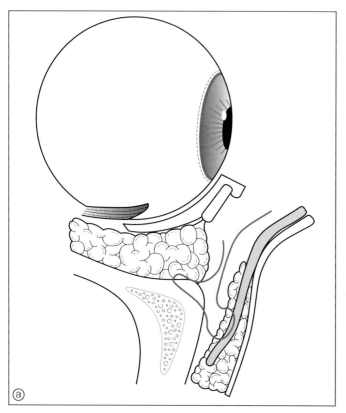

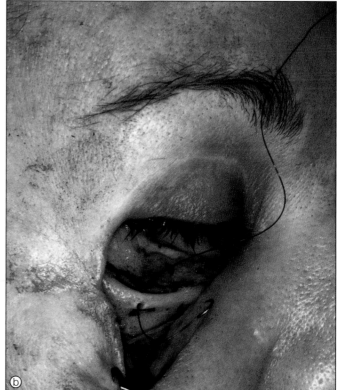

Figure 9.23 (a) Periosteal anchoring. (b) Application of drill hole.

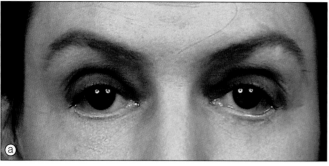

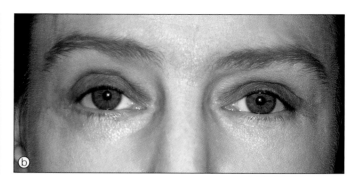

Figure 9.24 Before and after drill-hole fixation.

In retracted lids with very prominent eyes, insertion of a spacer is needed to lengthen the lid upward – now, most commonly, Alloderm is used (**Figs 9.25–9.28**).

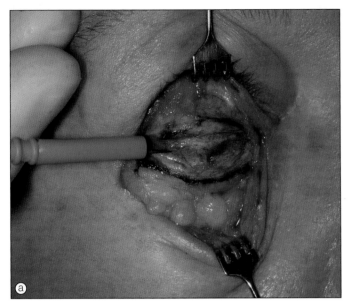 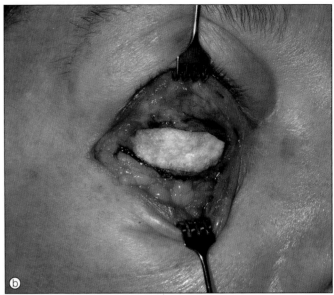

Figure 9.25 Insertion of spacer (Alloderm).

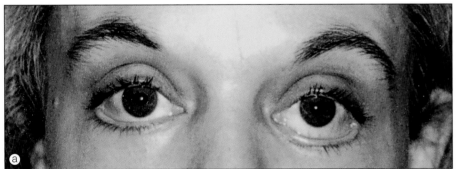

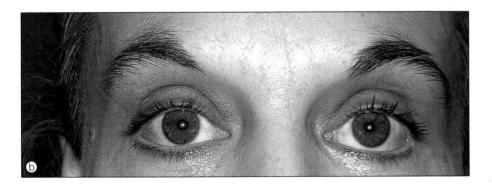

Figure 9.26 (a) A patient with prominent eyes and lower lid retraction. (b) After insertion of spacer.

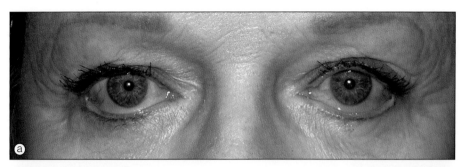

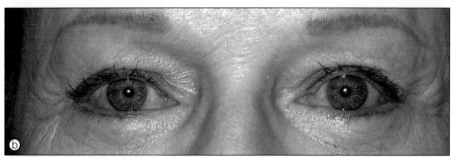

Figure 9.27 Correction by simple spacer insertion.

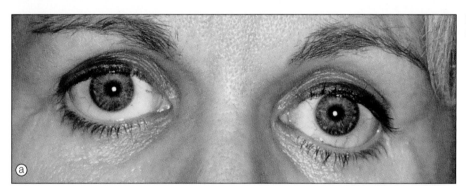

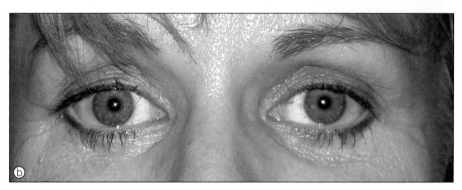

Figure 9.28 Correction by spacer insertion and secondary vertical cheeklift.

There is a higher revision rate in reconstructive cheeklift patients. Among 44 consecutive cases, 38% required more than one surgery and almost 10% required more than two operations.

To correct postoperative problems related to cheeklift, remember the mnemonic A-V-IS, or what it takes to ascend a tall peak like Mount Everest:

■ <u>a</u>nchoring;

■ <u>v</u>ertical recruitment; and

■ <u>i</u>nsertion of <u>s</u>pacer.

Laser Blepharoplasty of the Upper Eyelid

Chapter 10

Jemshed A Khan

Patient Selection

The goal of cosmetic upper eyelid blepharoplasty in the Caucasian patient is usually to improve appearance by reducing the gravitational and age-related redundancy, descent, and herniation of the upper eyelid tissues. One should examine and document common concurrent conditions including eyelid ptosis.

Patients should be carefully selected (**Figs 10.1 & 10.2**) with reference to the following:

- primary problem is redundant upper eyelid skin, orbicularis, and fat;
- no significant eyelid margin malposition;
- satisfactory eyebrow position; and
- satisfactory lacrimal gland position.

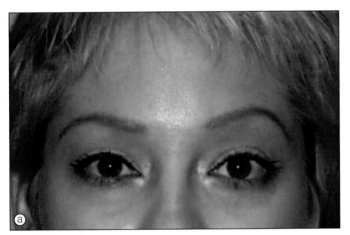

Figure 10.1 (a) Excellent candidate for upper eyelid blepharoplasty. Primary problem is isolated redundancy, descent, and herniation of the upper eyelid tissues.

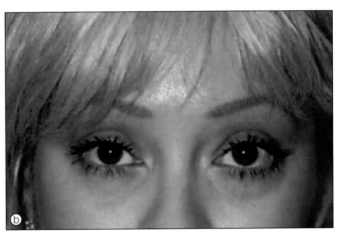

Figure 10.1 (b) Same patient after upper eyelid blepharoplasty.

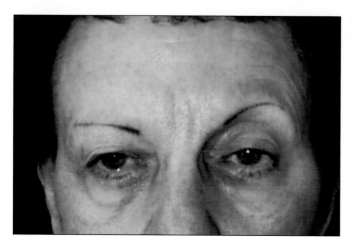

Figure 10.2 Poor candidate for upper eyelid blepharoplasty, given underlying eyebrow asymmetry and ptosis.

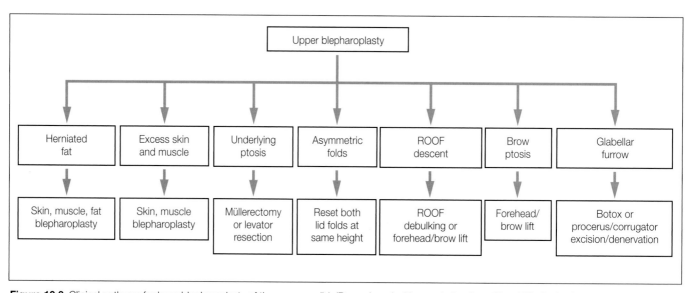

Figure 10.3 Clinical pathway for laser blepharoplasty of the upper eyelid. (Reproduced with permission from Chen WP. Oculoplastic surgery: the essentials. New York: Thieme; 2001: 176.)

The margin reflex distance (MRD) obtained with eyebrows manually raised (referred to as MRDb) is highly predictive of the post-blepharoplasty MRD. Balloting the globe while examining the superior sulcus helps determine which fat pads should be resected. Any pre-existing eyebrow ptosis, eyelid ptosis, or nasal webbing should be documented and emphasized to the patient (**Figs 10.4 & 10.5**). While the brows are manually raised, the superior sulcus is examined for evidence of herniating nasal and preaponeurotic fat pads and to search for lacrimal gland prolapse (**Fig. 10.6**). Finally, the extent of lateral hooding and retro-orbicularis oculi fat (ROOF) should be noted.

Search for lagophthalmos by having the patients passively close their eyelids as if sleeping or looking downward (**Fig. 10.7**). Slit-lamp corneal evaluation, rose bengal or fluorescein epithelial staining, or the Schirmer tear test help screen for dry-eye patients. An ocular examination including Bell's phenomenon testing may help document any pre-existing ophthalmic pathology. At this point, the surgeon should have a clear understanding of the patient's expectations, surgical risk factors, and underlying anatomic eyelid changes. With this information, the surgeon may now proceed to negotiate a surgical plan that safely meets the patient's needs and expectations.

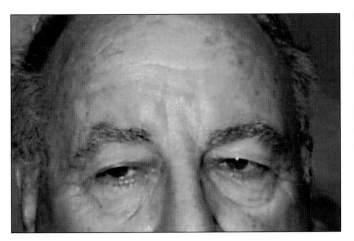

Figure 10.4 With the eyebrows in a normal position, one cannot determine from the margin reflex distance whether or not there is also an underlying eyelid ptosis.

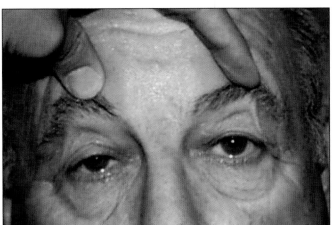

Figure 10.5 One can determine from the margin reflex distance obtained with eyebrows manually elevated – referred to as MRDb – that there is also a relative eyelid ptosis.

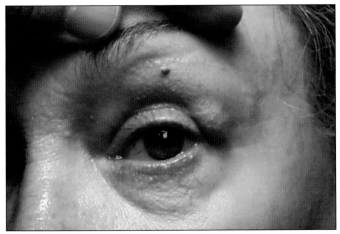

Figure 10.6 While the brows are manually raised, the superior sulcus is examined. Note evidence of herniating nasal fat pad and lacrimal gland prolapse.

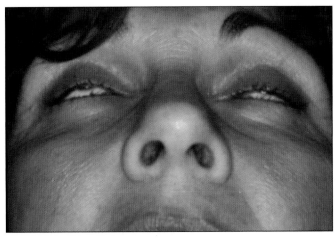

Figure 10.7 Demonstration of lagophthalmos.

Laser Instruments, Safety, Selection, and Parameters

Useful instruments include a millimeter ruler, 0.3mm toothed platform forceps, needle holder, stitch scissors, and hemostat. Metal eye shields and guards are needed. A bipolar or other cautery device is also necessary. Since there is a combustion hazard associated with CO_2 laser use, the patient should be draped with wet cloth towels. The superb hemostasis achieved by the CO_2 laser is due to the zone of coagulative and thermal injury created by the laser (**Fig. 10.8**).

Please see Chapter 11 for discussion of CO_2 laser parameters and laser safety.

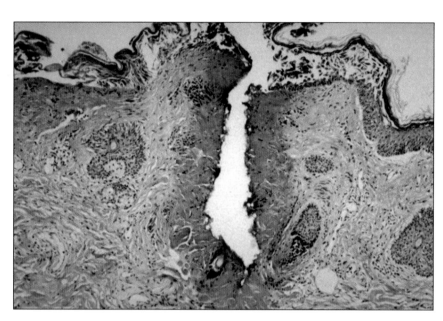

Figure 10.8 Histopathologic examination of CO_2 laser eyelid incision. Note the purple zone of thermal injury surrounding the laser-created tissue cleft, running vertically in this image. Image courtesy of Brian Biesman, MD.

CO_2 laser (10 600nm)

- Focused spot size of 0.3mm or less
- Wattage setting varies by manufacturer
- Continuous wave or pulsed setting
- Articulated arm beam delivery

Surgical Steps

1. Mark the proposed upper eyelid crease

When marking the eyelid skin for excision, always remember that the inferior border of the skin incision usually becomes the postoperative eyelid crease. If the inferior incisions are misplaced or asymmetrical, then the final results will be askew. Therefore, careful initial skin markings are critical. In Caucasian eyelids, the inferior incision is usually marked 9–11mm superior to the central eyelid margin, 4mm superior to the upper punctum, and 6mm superior to the lateral canthal angle (**Figs 10.9 & 10.10**). These markings need to be lower in Asian eyelids. The female eyelid usually has a higher arched crease compared with the male eyelid. (In the Asian eyelid, be certain that the incision height and curvature is a natural extension of any pre-existing epicanthal folds.) The eyelid crease (and inferior marking) usually curves somewhat downwards as it extends towards the medial canthus and lateral canthus.

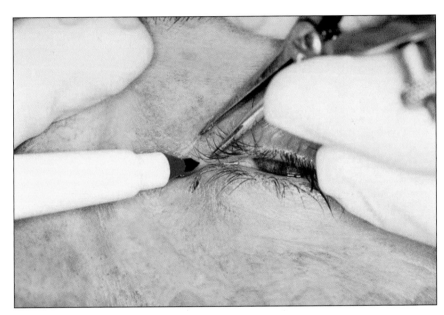

Figure 10.9 An inked millimeter calibrated caliper is used to mark the medial aspect of the lower eyelid crease 4mm superior to the punctum.

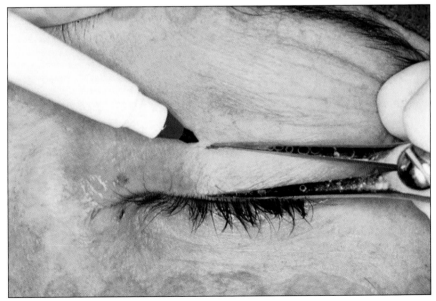

Figure 10.10 An inked millimeter calibrated caliper is used to mark the central aspect of the lower eyelid crease 9–11mm superior to the eyelid margin.

2. Determine the safe amount of skin removal with pinch technique

Perfectly symmetrical skin markings are the foundation upon which the success of the remainder of the operation rests. Any asymmetry will carry forward in the operation and adversely affect the final outcome. With the patient supine, determine the amount of skin removal using pinch or other techniques (**Fig. 10.11**). While pinching, be certain that the lids can passively close (**Fig. 10.12**). This should prevent postoperative lagophthalmos due to excessive skin removal. The medial extent of removal is superior to the punctum but should be moved laterally when there is a tendency to medial canthal webbing. The tendency towards medial webbing may be determined preoperatively: gently pinch the lateral walls of the nasal bridge and tug inferiorly. By observing the medial canthal area for webbing during this maneuver, one can judge the tendency to webbing. The lateral extent of removal is often determined by hooding and may be limited by the lateral orbital rim. Ink the margins for resection and then remeasure with calipers to ensure perfect symmetry. A pinch forcep is shown in **Figure 10.13**.

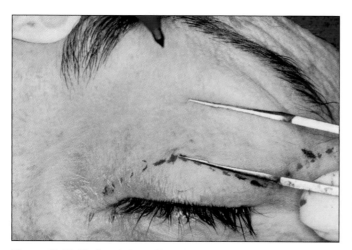

Figure 10.11 Pinch technique. The inferior jaw of the forceps engages the inferior skin mark.

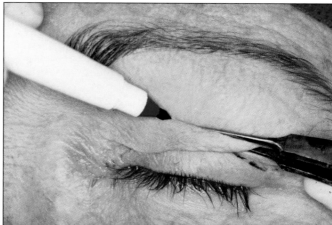

Figure 10.12 Redundant skin is gathered between the forceps jaws. Care is taken that no lagophthalmos is induced, and the superior resection margin is inked.

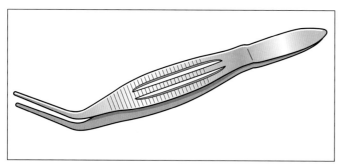

Figure 10.13 Specially designed ambidextrous 'Khan Ink and Pinch' forceps for blepharoplasty skin marking. Note square atraumatic jaws are offset from the forceps' shafts to allow gathering of redundant skin. Minute tip serrations engage the inferior crease. Calibrated millimeter markings help ensure symmetry (Courtesy of Storz Instrument Company, St Louis, MO, USA).

3. Expose the orbital septum

Local anesthesia with optional intravenous sedation provides adequate patient comfort for blepharoplasty. Sublingual diazepam (5.0mg tablet) helps reduce anxiety when the procedure is performed entirely under local anesthesia. The local anesthetic consists of 2% lidocaine hydrochloride (Xylocaine with epinephrine 1:200 000) mixed 1:1 with 0.75% bupivicaine hydrochloride (Marcaine). For better diffusion of anesthetic, hyaluronidase (Wydase) is often added.

Approximately 1.5–2.0mL of anesthetic solution is injected subcutaneously via a 30-gauge needle into the mid-portion of each eyelid. The raised subcutaneous bleb of anesthetic is then digitally massaged medially and laterally. Waiting 10 to 20 minutes allows the epinephrine to create a hemostatic effect (**Fig. 10.14**).

When incising the skin and orbicularis, be very careful of the levator aponeurosis, which may be directly beneath the orbicularis at the inferior incision (**Fig. 10.15**).

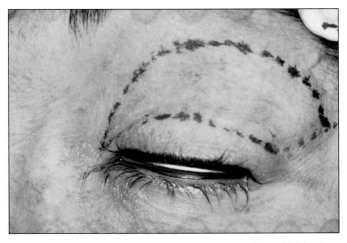

Figure 10.14 Final appearance of skin marked for excision with injection applied.

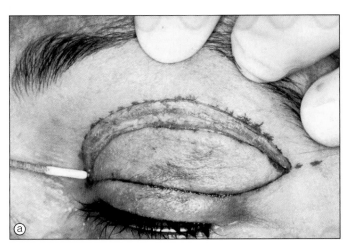

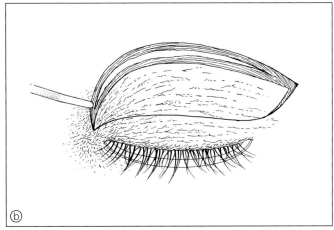

Figure 10.15 Left upper eyelid. Incision of the skin and orbicularis. Keep the beam perpendicular to the skin surface and repeat passes with wound gently spread until through the orbicularis. Note the distinctive reddish-brown color of the orbicularis muscle, and the pale septum visible between the divided orbicularis edges. Be very careful of the levator aponeurosis, which may be directly beneath the orbicularis at the inferior incision.

This author usually excises skin and orbicularis as a single specimen, but separate layered excision is also acceptable. When excising the skin–muscle ellipse, apply strong traction and counter-traction while developing the surgical plane. Stay in the plane of the post-orbicularis fascia, being careful to avoid transecting the levator inferiorly (**Figs 10.16 & 10.17**).

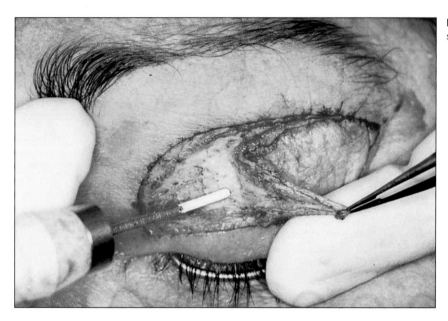

Figure 10.16 Left upper eyelid. Laser excision of the skin–muscle ellipse.

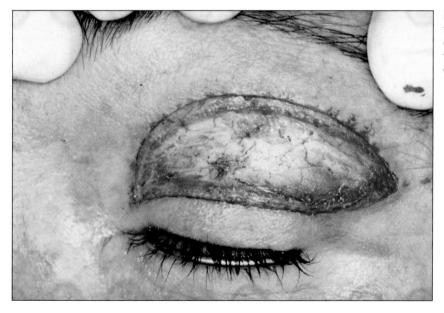

Figure 10.17 Left upper eyelid following excision of the skin–muscle ellipse. Note the clean surgical dissection with minimal hemorrhage. The expanse of the orbital septum is clearly visible, as are the orbicularis edges.

4. Incise the septum

It is important to free each of the fat pads from any encumbering structures. Specifically, the overlying orbital septum must be divided for each fat pad before the fat can be prolapsed. The orbital septum is opened laterally or medially. Buttonhole the septum until fat prolapses freely. It is often helpful to ballot the globe in order to inspect and visualize the underlying preaponeurotic (postseptal) fat pocket (**Fig. 10.18**). The entire horizontal width of the exposed septum is then divided (**Fig. 10.19**).

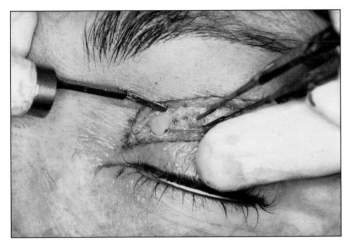

Figure 10.18 Left upper eyelid. Buttonhole the orbital septum laterally or nasally. As much as possible, keep the laser pointed tangential or away from the globe. Ballot the globe and inspect to visualize the underlying postseptal fat pocket. Buttonhole the septum until fat prolapses freely.

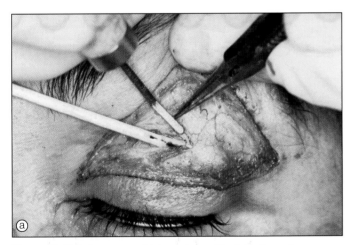

Figure 10.19 Left upper eyelid. Laser is used to divide the entire horizontal width of the exposed septum over a backstop such as a dripping wet cotton-tip applicator or metal guard.

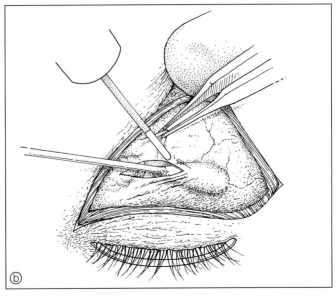

Be sure to identify the exposed upper eyelid fat pad and underlying levator muscle. Grasp the fat pad with forceps and bluntly strip it free of the levator muscle and aponeurosis (**Fig. 10.20**). Excise the fat pad to the level of the orbital rim or Whitnall's ligament. The fat pad may be excised across a closed hemostat, or divided against a backstop. Avoid the lacrimal gland laterally (**Fig. 10.21**). Adequate hemostasis is important because of the caliber of vessels associated with the fat pocket.

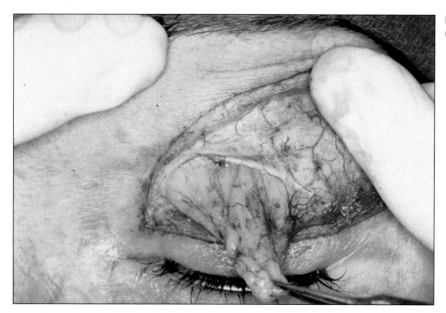

Figure 10.20 Left upper eyelid. Identify the exposed upper eyelid fat pad and underlying levator muscle.

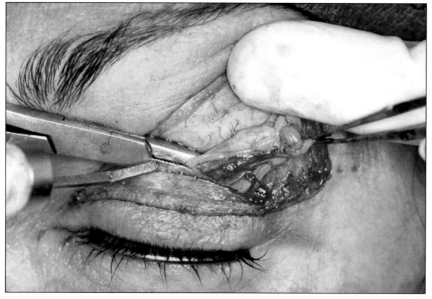

Figure 10.21 Excision of the preaponeurotic fat pad.

5. Mobilize and excise the nasal fat pad

Gently spread the fascia over the nasal fat pad with hemostats. Ballot the globe to bring the fat pad forward. Make an 'X'-shaped incision over the nasal fat pad. Deepen the incision until fat prolapses (**Fig. 10.22**). Grasp and immobilize the protruding knuckle of fat and then use a cotton-tip applicator to bluntly strip away tissues retaining the nasal fat pad (**Fig. 10.23**). The base of the nasal fat pad usually requires supplemental local anesthesia injection for pain control. The fat pad may be excised across a closed hemostat, or divided against a backstop. Again, adequate hemostasis is important because of the caliber of vessels associated with the fat pocket (**Fig. 10.24**).

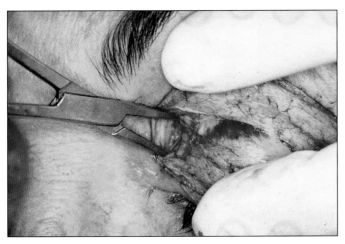

Figure 10.22 Left upper eyelid. Hemostat jaws are used to spread the fascia over the nasal fat pad. The globe is then balloted to bring the fat pad forward. An 'X'-shaped incision is made over the nasal fat pad and deepened until fat prolapses.

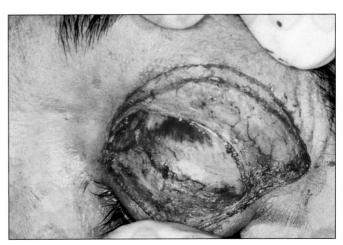

Figure 10.24 Appearance of surgical field following fat pad excision. Note the levator muscle and aponeurosis, as well as the retro-orbicularis oculi fat (ROOF) tissues overlying the orbital rim.

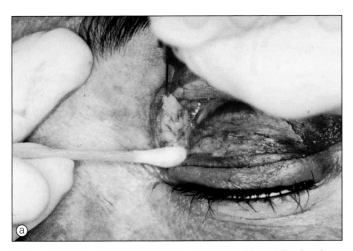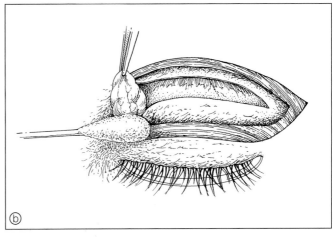

Figure 10.23 The prolapsing fat pad is grasped and immobilized and a cotton-tip applicator is used to bluntly strip away tissues retaining the nasal fat pad. The wound is inspected for residual fat.

6. Excision of ROOF if necessary

At times, retro-orbicularis oculi fat may be prominent and may be excised. This is usually helpful in patients with thick redundant tissues obscuring the lateral half of the orbital rim (**Figs 10.25 & 10.26**). To excise ROOF, grasp the orbicularis of the upper wound edge. Trim the orbicularis and underlying ROOF flush with the skin edge. Reflect the ROOF from the deep connective tissue overlying the orbital rim (**Fig. 10.27**). Do not expose bare periosteum because the skin may become adherent after surgery (**Fig. 10.28**). Cauterize any bleeders.

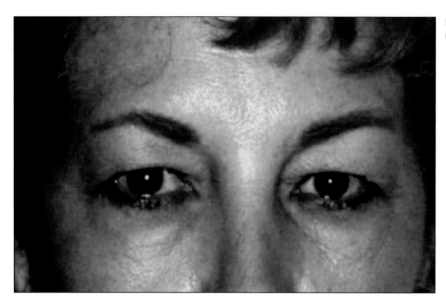

Figure 10.25 Candidate for retro-orbicularis oculi fat (ROOF) excision. Note the redundant lateral tissue.

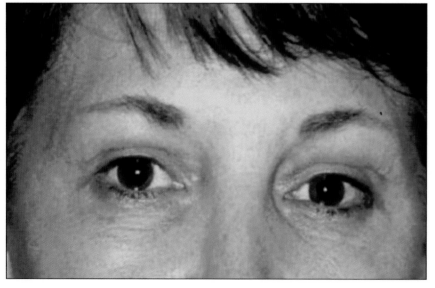

Figure 10.26 Patient following retro-orbicularis oculi fat (ROOF) excision. Note the definition of the lateral superior orbital rims.

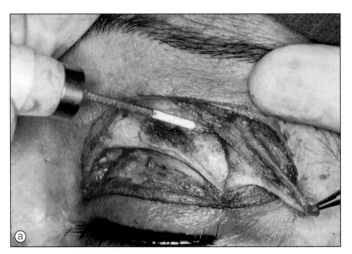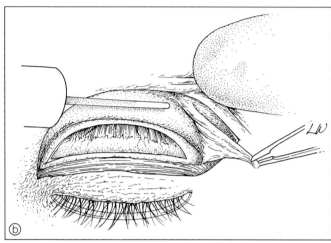

Figure 10.27 The retro-orbicularis oculi fat (ROOF) tissue is reflected in the avascular supra-periosteal plane over the lateral half of the superior orbital rim.

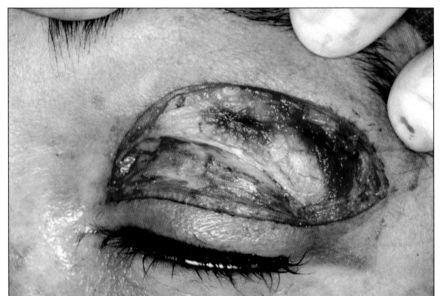

Figure 10.28 Care is taken to spare a layer of loose tissue overlying the periosteum.

7. Closure of incision

Close the skin incision with interrupted 6-0 Prolene nasally and running 6-0 Prolene for the remainder. Take only superficial dermal bites (0.5mm depth) to reduce bleeding. Other options include recreating the eyelid crease by placing three stitches through the dermis of the lower skin edge and then through the surface of the levator aponeurosis along the superior tarsal border to the upper skin edge. Deeper (1.5mm depth) bites are taken lateral to the outer canthal angle to prevent dehiscence. Use a taper needle to reduce bleeding. Ointment is applied to the incision as well as the inferior cul-de-sac if the patient is not blinking fully. Stitches are left in for 7–15 days.

Postoperative instructions include frequent ice packs, erythromycin ophthalmic ointment to the incision once daily, and avoiding strenuous activity.

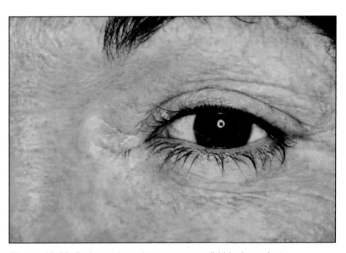

Figure 10.29 Patient prior to laser upper eyelid blepharoplasty.

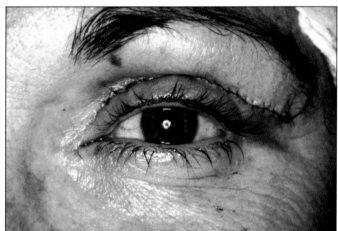

Figure 10.30 Same patient immediately following laser upper eyelid blepharoplasty with retro-orbicularis oculi fat (ROOF) tissue excision.

CO$_2$ Laser Transconjunctival Blepharoplasty

Chapter 11

Jemshed A Khan

Patient Selection

Transconjunctival laser blepharoplasty is a useful technique for addressing lower eyelid fat pad herniation (**Fig. 11.1**). Compared with other approaches, the transconjunctival technique avoids any cutaneous stitches or incisions, disrupts neither the orbicularis layer nor its motor innervation, and affords a remarkably brief convalescence.

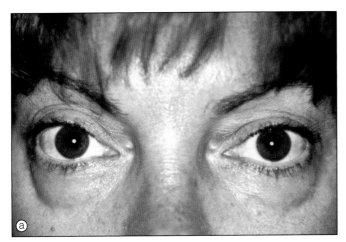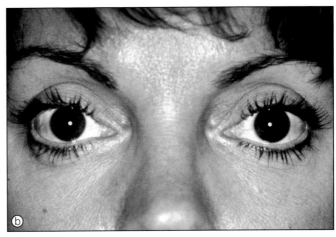

Figure 11.1 (a) Excellent candidate for transconjunctival blepharoplasty. Primary problem is isolated to lower eyelid fat pad herniation. (b) Same patient following transconjunctival blepharoplasty.

The transconjunctival technique does not address common concurrent eyelid conditions such as eyelid laxity, wrinkles, festoons, malar edema and folds, and suborbicularis oculi fat (SOOF) descent (**Fig. 11.2**). The transconjunctival approach may be combined with other procedures to address any of the previously listed concurrent conditions, and may be modified to allow repositioning of the lower eyelid fat pads to address tear trough deformities (**Fig. 11.3**).

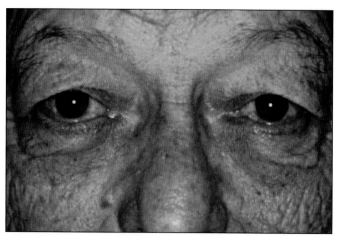

Figure 11.2 Poor candidate for transconjunctival blepharoplasty, given significant eyelid wrinkles and festoons.

Patient selection for laser transconjunctival blepharoplasty of the lower lid should be based on:

- primary problem is lower eyelid fat pad herniation
- no significant eyelid margin malposition
- satisfactory lower eyelid skin without significant wrinkling
- satisfactory midface continuum

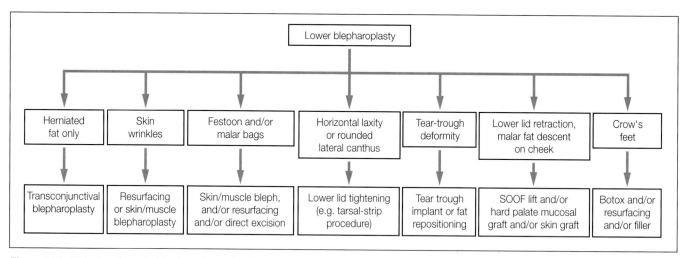

Figure 11.3 Clinical pathway for blepharoplasty of the lower eyelid.

Laser Selection and Parameters

Incisional CO_2 lasers suitable for blepharoplasty are available from several manufacturers, including Lumenis (formerly the medical laser division of Coherent Inc. and Sharplan/ESC) and Nidek. Each company uses a slightly different CO_2 delivery system, and actual incisional parameters vary accordingly. A small spot size of 0.3mm or less is important to reduce the zone of thermal injury. CO_2 lasers that use a hollow waveguide rather than an articulated arm to transmit the beam from the laser tube to the hand piece are not as popular because the exit beam is divergent rather than coherent, collimated, and focused (**Figs 11.4 & 11.5**). Appropriate formal didactic training in laser blepharoplasty and laser safety is essential and is beyond the scope of this chapter. For further information, see References 1 and 2.

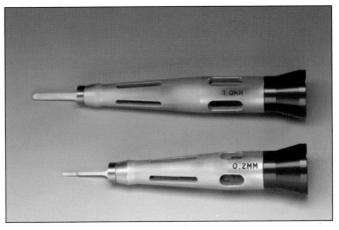

Figure 11.5 Focused hand-piece. The focused hand-piece converts the collimated output of the articulated arm into a smaller and more intense focused spot that is used to divide tissue.

Parameters of CO_2 laser (10 600nm)

- Focused spot size of 0.3mm or less
- Wattage setting varies by manufacturer
- Continuous-wave or pulsed setting
- Articulated-arm beam delivery

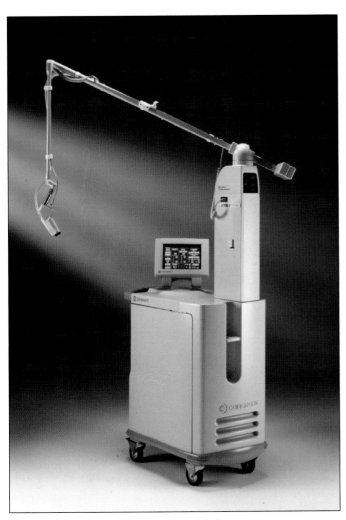

Figure 11.4 Articulated arm. The rigid articulated arm of the UltraPulse CO_2 laser delivers focused, collimated, and coherent laser energy to the hand piece.

Laser Safety

Laser safety is crucial because of the numerous hazards associated with unsafe handling techniques (**Fig. 11.6**). The surgeon must acquire appropriate knowledge, motor skills, and laser-safe instrumentation before embarking upon laser blepharoplasty (**Fig. 11.7, Table 11.1**). For further information, see Reference 3.

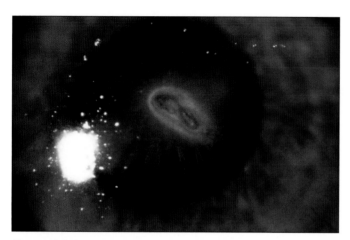

Figure 11.6 Corneal injury caused by CO_2 laser during blepharoplasty procedure.

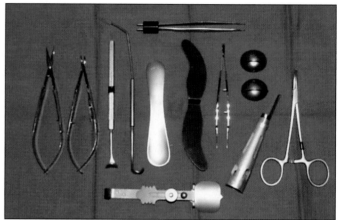

Figure 11.7 Safety instruments used during CO_2 laser blepharoplasty have an antireflective finish. Instruments (left to right) include Wescott scissors, micro needle holder, pair of matte-finish Desmarres retractors, modified Khan–Jaeger laser eyelid plate, 'propeller' laser backstop, Castroviejo 0.5mm platform tying forceps, pair of metal scleral guards, laser handpiece, and hemostat. Top: bipolar cautery forceps. Bottom: laser blepharoplasty clamp.

Table 11.1: Safety issues for laser blepharoplasty.	
Globe protection	Metal interpositional shield or scleral shield
Tissue protection	Metal backstop or hemostat
Appropriate laser, laser settings, and laser focus	
Laser reflection hazard	Anti-reflection treatment of metal instruments
Combustion hazard	Use wet drapes
Operator smoke hazard	Use smoke evacuator and laser masks
Operator ocular hazard	Wear wavelength-appropriate laser-safe goggles
Governmental standards	Follow OSHA and State standards

Anatomic Landmarks

The location of the inferior oblique muscle should be clearly envisioned prior to embarking upon transconjunctival blepharoplasty. The inferior oblique is reliably located in the cleft or separation between the nasal and central fat pads (**Fig. 11.8**). The inferior oblique muscle originates from the periosteum adjacent to the proximal bony nasolacrimal duct and passes inferior to the nasal fat pad and superior to the central fat pad. Arising from the inferior oblique is an expansion of connective tissue that sometimes restrains the contiguous fat of the central and lateral fat pads. This tissue, termed the *arcuate expansion*, may be divided if necessary (**Fig. 11.9**).

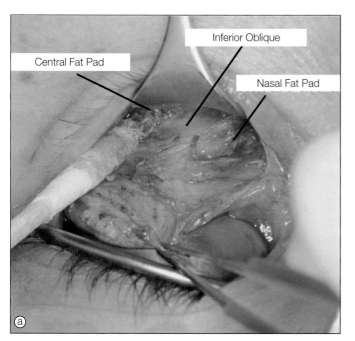

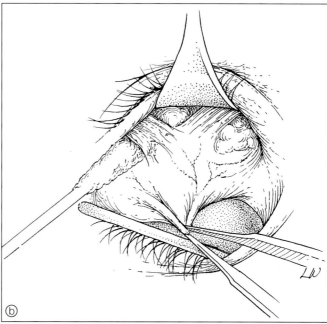

Figure 11.8 Inferior oblique muscle is reliably located in the cleft or separation between the nasal and central fat pads.

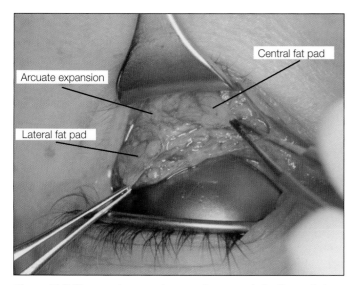

Figure 11.9 The arcuate expansion sometimes constrains the central and temporal fat pads.

Clinical pearls

- Recommended instruments (Storz Instrument Company, St Louis, MO, USA) include a Khan–Jaeger laser eyelid plate, Castroviejo 0.5mm toothed platform tying forceps, Desmarres retractor (dull finish), bipolar cautery, hemostat (fine curved), and protective metal scleral contact lens.

- The inferior oblique can always be located between the nasal and central fat pads.

- If the fat is restrained between the central and lateral fat pads, look for and divide the anteriorly located fibrous band of tissue (arcuate expansion).

- The lateral fat pad is easier to remove once separated from the underlying lower eyelid retractor.

Surgical Steps

1. Prolapse the inferior fat pads and fornix

Adequate prolapse and exposure of the conjunctival fornix is an essential prelude to successful transconjunctival incision (**Fig. 11.10**). The key to this step is to ballot the globe so as to prolapse the fat and conjunctiva anteriorly whilst simultaneously having the assistant retract the lower eyelid margin with two fingers. Retraction of the lower eyelid margin requires that the pads of the assistant's fingers be placed directly upon the eyelid margin itself in order to exert sufficient inferior traction. When performed successfully, a liberal horizontal roll of prolapsing fat and overlying conjunctiva will present itself quite reliably and visibly. The use of the titanium Khan–Jaeger plate allows one to ballot the globe posteriorly in order to prolapse the fat anteriorly while also protecting the globe.

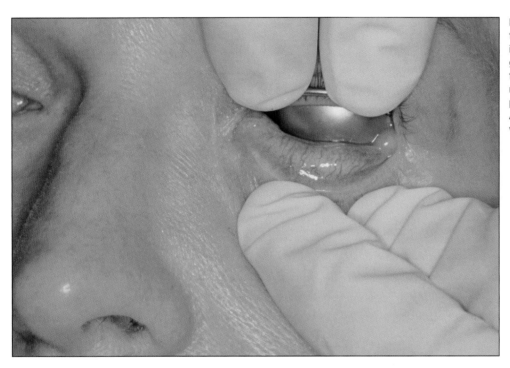

Figure 11.10 Demonstration of proper technique for fully prolapsing the inferior fornix. Note ballottement of globe and positioning of assistant's fingers on the eyelid margin. Globe may be balloted posteriorly with Jaeger plate or metal scleral contact lens. Assistant retracts lower eyelid margin with two fingers.

2. Incise the conjunctiva

Conjunctival incision placement is important in order to efficiently expose the three underlying fat pads while avoiding unintended injury to surrounding structures. The medial landmark for incision placement is the inferior border of the lateral tip of the caruncle. The incision is carried laterally, staying 4mm inferior to the tarsus and to where it curves towards the lateral canthal angle (**Fig. 11.11**).

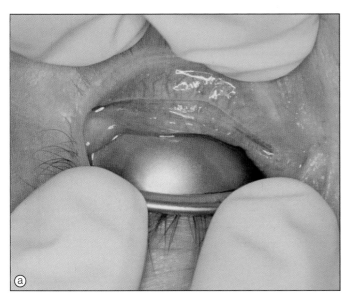 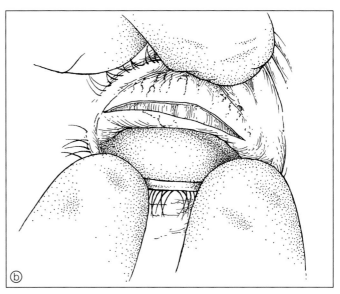

Figure 11.11 Incision originates from the inferior border of the caruncle, continues laterally 4.0mm inferior to the lower edge of the tarsal plate, and extends to the lateral canthal angle (left lower lid).

Essential steps

When incising the conjunctiva:

■ Begin at the inferior border of the lateral tip of the caruncle

■ Continue laterally

■ Stay 4mm below the base of the tarsal plate

■ Continue to within 2mm of the lateral canthal angle

■ Angle the beam towards the inferior orbital rim

3. Expose the orbital septum

After carrying the incision deeper until it spreads open, one may either continue the incision deeper while angling towards the orbital rim, or bluntly dissect the orbicularis off the orbital septum with a cotton-tip applicator (**Fig. 11.12**). With the former approach, one will often times automatically expose the three fat pads of the lower eyelid, in which case one may proceed to Step 5. It is still advisable to divide the lateral fat pad from the underlying lower eyelid retractors.

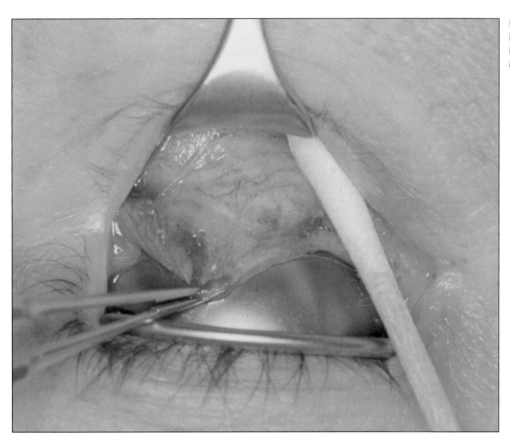

Figure 11.12 Spread incision. The incision is deepened with the laser until it can be spread open with a cotton-tip applicator.

Essential steps

To expose the orbital septum:

- Carry the incision deeper *until it spreads open*, exposing the septum

- Place a Desmarres retractor

- Grasp the inferior conjunctival wound edge with 0.5mm toothed forceps

- Spread the wound farther open by sweeping a cotton-tip inferiorly across the septum

4. Incise the septum over the nasal, central, and lateral fat pads

It is important to free each of the fat pads from any encumbering structures. Specifically, the overlying orbital septum must be divided for each fat pad before the fat can prolapse freely (**Fig. 11.13**). The lateral fat pad may be more difficult to mobilize because the overlying septum may be adherent to the inferior lateral orbital rim.

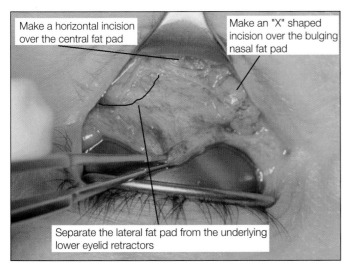

Make a horizontal incision over the central fat pad

Make an "X" shaped incision over the bulging nasal fat pad

Separate the lateral fat pad from the underlying lower eyelid retractors

Figure 11.13 Separate incisions are placed over each fat pad of the lower left eyelid.

Nasal fat pad

- Ballot the globe to bring the fat pad forward
- Make an 'X'-shaped incision over the nasal fat pad
- Deepen the incision until fat prolapses

Central fat pad

- Ballot the globe to bring the fat pad forward
- Make a horizontal 10–12mm incision over the central fat pad
- Place the incision 2–3mm superior to the inferior orbital rim
- Deepen the incision until fat prolapses

Lateral fat pad

- Expose the lateral fat pad
- Divide the fat pad from the underlying lower eyelid retractors
- Incise the overlying orbital septum
- Divide the arcuate expansion if necessary (fibrous anterior band separating the central and lateral fat pads)

5. Mobilize each fat pad

Nasal and central fat pads

The nasal and central fat pads generally prolapse quite easily (**Figs 11.14 & 11.15**). It is important to be aware of large vessels in the base of the nasal fat pad. An encircling fibrous band is often found at the base of the nasal fat pad and may be bluntly stripped away. The inferior oblique muscle may be reliably located along the inferior and lateral edge of the nasal fat pad.

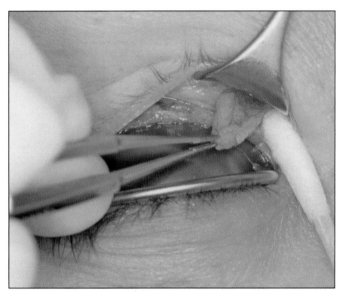

Figure 11.14 The nasal fat pad is mobilized with forceps and cotton-tip applicator.

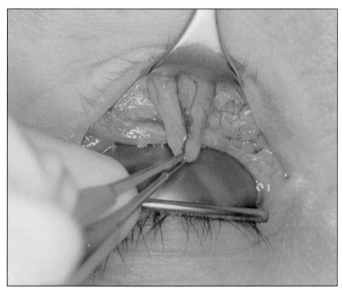

Figure 11.15 The central fat pad is mobilized through a horizontal incision.

Nasal fat pad

- Base of nasal fat pad may require supplemental local anesthesia injection
- Do NOT tug anteriorly on the fat pad
- Use a cotton-tip to strip away tissues retaining the nasal fat pad

Central fat pad

- Grasp prolapsing fat with forceps
- Do NOT tug anteriorly on the fat pad
- Use a cotton-tip to strip away tissues retaining the inferior aspect of the central fat pad

Lateral fat pad

The lateral fat pad is the most difficult to mobilize because it is adherent to the lower eyelid retractors and covered by a sometimes thick septum that is densely adherent to the inferior lateral rim (**Fig. 11.16**). Exposure is further compromised by the lateral canthal tendon. In the lateral aspect of the lateral pad there are often blood vessels that may bleed profusely. Therefore, exposure is maximized by excising any dense overlying septum and also freeing the fat pad from the underlying lower eyelid retractors. Even when properly mobilized, a deeper pad or further lateral fat may only become evident after first removing the presenting lateral fat and balloting the globe.

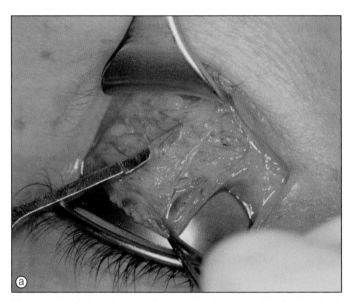
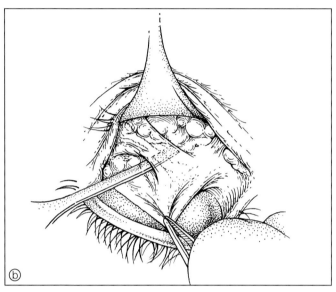

Figure 11.16 (a & b) The arcuate expansion is a fibrous band obscuring the tip of the underlying laser probe.

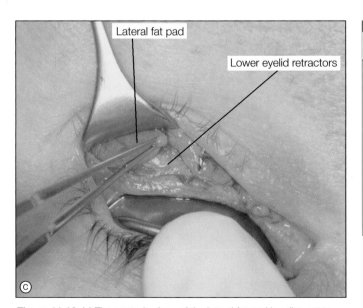

Lateral fat pad

Lower eyelid retractors

Figure 11.16 (c) The posterior face of the lateral fat pad is adherent to the lower eyelid retractors.

Essential steps

- The lateral fat may come out in two layers
- The lateral fat pad is adherent to the underlying lower eyelid retractors
- Sharply divide the lateral fat pad from the underlying retractors
- The lateral pad may be restrained by the arcuate expansion
- Divide the arcuate expansion if necessary

6. Divide each fat pad flush with the orbital rim

Nasal and central fat pads

One can achieve remarkable postoperative lower eyelid symmetry by using the symmetric positions of the paired inferior orbital rims. Therefore, it is important to use the bony inferior orbital rim as the sole landmark when deciding exactly where to transect the herniating lower eyelid fat. One can grasp the herniating fat with a hemostat which rests upon the orbital rim. Thus assured, one can proceed with excision of the fat. Other methods include piecemeal excision of the protruding fat. After excising the protruding fat, it is important to immediately ballot and see if any more fat comes forward easily.

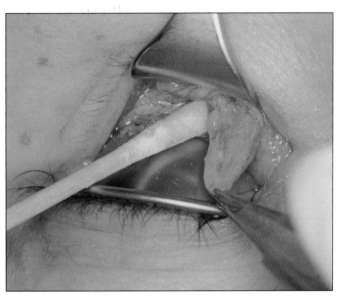

Figure 11.17 Demonstration of a moist cotton-tip applicator employed as a backstop for laser division of the nasal fat pad.

Essential steps

- Transect each fat pad flush with the inferior orbital rim
- Use a metal Desmarres retractor, moist cotton-tip, or hemostat as a backstop
- The central fat pad prolapses easily and generally presents little difficulty

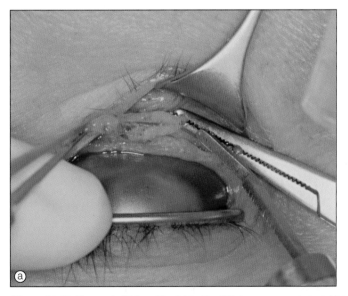
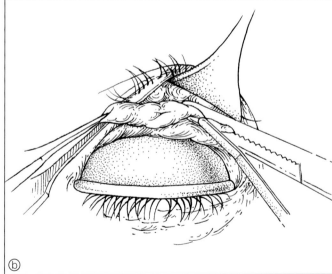

Figure 11.18 The central fat pad is divided by CO_2 laser over a clamped hemostat.

Lateral fat pad

Positioning a hemostat properly in the tight lateral area requires diligence and experience. It is not uncommon to find that more fat prolapses immediately following the first excision. Also, there may still be a residual temporal bulge of fat that requires further division of the septum. Therefore, assiduousness and patience are necessary to achieve adequate temporal fat excision (**Fig. 11.19**).

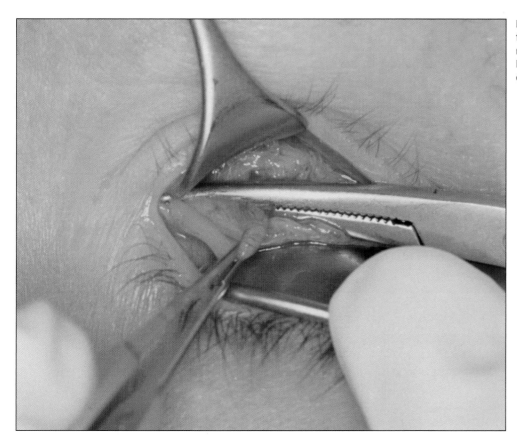

Figure 11.19 The lateral fat pad is transected flush with the inferior orbital rim and requires use of a metal Desmarres retractor, moist cotton-tip, or hemostat as a backstop.

7. Reposition the eyelid and ballot to look for any residual bulging fat

Balloting is an important final step. Often, one may find residual fat that was overlooked earlier in the procedure (**Fig. 11.20**). Such fat may not come forward until later in the procedure because it had been constrained by cautery or clamping of the overlying fat.

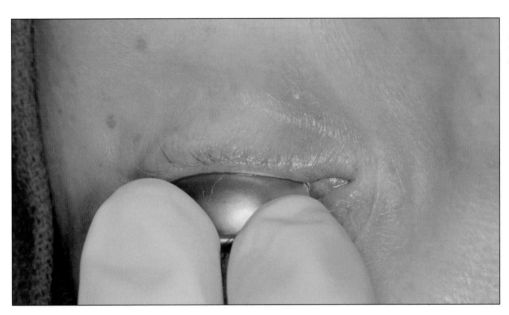

Figure 11.20 Finger pressure is applied to the protective shield in order to retropulse the globe and prolapse forward any residual excess fat.

Essential steps

- Ballot by applying firm pressure against the globe
- Examine the contours of both lower eyelids
- Look for any bulging or asymmetry
- Excise further fat as needed
- Look for and cauterize any bleeding points

8. Closure

Postoperatively, the patient is instructed to:

1. avoid significant lifting or straining for several days

2. heed written instructions that include the warning signs of retrobulbar hemorrhage

3. use antibiotic ointment, which is applied to the inferior fornix each evening

4. avoid contact lenses for 1 week

5. use icepacks for 7 days

6. elevate the head of the bed, when sleeping, for 1 week.

Oral and topical corticosteroids are prescribed only when patients develop significant postoperative chemosis or eyelid edema. Patients are generally seen 9 to 14 days following surgery.

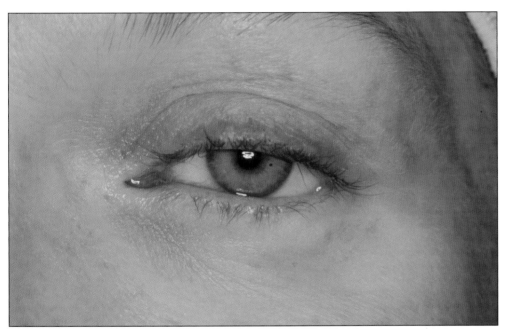

Figure 11.21 Appearance at end of procedure.

Essential steps

- Tug upwards on the eyelid to prevent inversion or overriding of the wound
- No suture is used
- Remove eye shield
- Place ointment
- Reassure patient

REFERENCES

1. Khan JA. Introduction of laser incisional surgery. In: Biesman B, ed. Lasers in facial aesthetic and reconstructive surgery. Baltimore, MD: William & Wilkins; 1998:91–7.

2. Biesman BS, Khan JA. Laser incisional surgery. Clin Plast Surg 2000;27:213–20.

3. Khan JA, Biesman B. Carbon dioxide laser physics, laser tissue interaction, and laser Safety. In: Biesman B, ed. Lasers in facial aesthetic and reconstructive surgery. Baltimore, MD: Williams & Wilkins; 1998:1–13.

Ptosis (Blepharoptosis)

Chapter 12

William PD Chen

Traditionally, ptosis has been divided into either the congenital or acquired category. In the literature there have been publications reporting a 90% preponderance of congenital ptosis versus acquired ptosis; and yet there have also been papers reporting that acquired ptosis constituted the majority of cases. Obviously, the reported incidence will depend heavily on the type of patients profiled by the observers, their training and subspecialty inclination, their referral pattern, and even the town that they practice in (whether it is a younger population). This method of classification does not immediately yield any clue as to the origin of the particular type of ptosis, although it tends generally to fall into those with poor to fair levator function (congenital ptosis), and those with good levator function (acquired ptosis). In this classification, the most prevalent form of ptosis to be encountered in a clinical ophthalmologist's practice would be involutional ptosis ('senile' ptosis) within the acquired ptosis group. The etiology of this form of ptosis would include aging, stretching of the levator aponeurotic complex, as well as postsurgical.

A more informative etiological classification deriving from the above is to categorize ptosis into the following groups:

- aponeurotic ptosis (from levator aponeurotic dehiscence or rarefaction);
- myogenic ptosis;
- neurogenic ptosis; and
- mechanical ptosis.

In this scheme, the traditional 'acquired ptosis' would fall into the involutional aponeurotic dehiscence type, while 'congenital ptosis' would be part of the myogenic group.

Aponeurotic ptosis would include involutional ptosis seen in elderly patients, where the levator aponeurosis (**Fig. 12.1**) may have undergone rarefaction or partial dehiscence along the superior tarsal border, resulting in elongation of the length of the muscle and a ptotic upper lid margin.

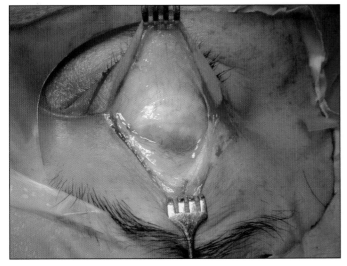

Figure 12.1 Open-sky view of levator aponeurosis and Whitnall's suspensory ligament, right upper lid.

Clinical findings in involutional ptosis may include mild to moderate ptosis, a high lid crease, and a good to excellent levator function (greater than 10mm). The clinician may be able to see the outline of the cornea through the upper lid skin when the patients close their eyelids. Intraoperatively, one may see fatty infiltration and degenerative changes of the levator aponeurosis, partial dehiscence of the medial portion of the levator muscle (**Fig. 12.2**), and lateral shifting of the tarsal plate (**Fig. 12.3**).

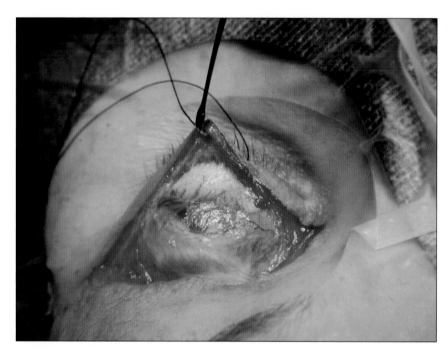

Figure 12.2 Dehiscence and fatty degeneration of the medial portion of the levator muscle in a left upper eyelid.

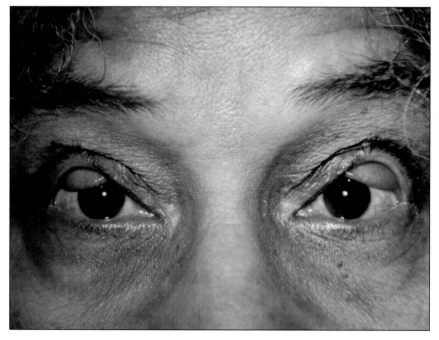

Figure 12.3 Lateral migration of the tarsi in an elderly woman.

Other causes include surgical trauma (ocular surgery, vitreoretinal surgery, enucleation, and evisceration), repeated subclinical injury to the upper lids (including contact lens wear and recurrent periorbital swelling), and actual traumatic injury.

Myogenic ptosis includes the broad category of congenital ptosis, congenital ptosis with superior rectus weakness (double elevator palsy), Marcus Gunn jaw winking ptosis, blepharophimosis, myasthenia gravis, chronic progressive external ophthalmoplegia, and rarer entities like muscular dystrophy.

Congenital ptosis typically presents at birth (**Fig. 12.4**). It is thought to be an isolated dystrophy of the levator muscle, at times manifesting as a hypoplasia of the muscle. On clinical examination the patient may present with mild to severe ptosis, and levator function in the poor (0–5mm) to fair (5–10mm) range. The eyelid typically shows absence of lid crease and may manifest lagophthalmos on downgaze. There is frequently a history from the parent that the child's eyelids do not approximate at night during sleep, although the cornea may be rolled up from an intact oculocephalic reflex (Bell's phenomenon). It may be unilateral or bilateral, with asymmetric involvement.

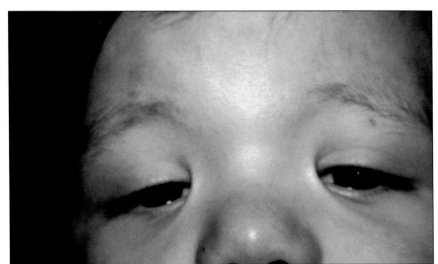

Figure 12.4 Congenital ptosis of the right upper lid. Note absence of crease on affected lid.

Marcus Gunn jaw winking ptosis (**Fig. 12.5a**) is a peculiar condition where the patient's ptosis appears to be lessened when the subject moves his or her lower jaw to the opposite side of the involved eyelid (**Fig. 12.5b**). For example, a patient who has ptosis of the right upper lid may reduce his ptosis when his jaw is moved laterally to the left side, or the patient may show fluctuation of his upper lid's ptotic position as he is having his meals (activating his masticatory muscles innervated by the fifth nerve). It is thought to be an aberrant innervational connection between the levator and the fifth nerve, although the exact location is unclear.

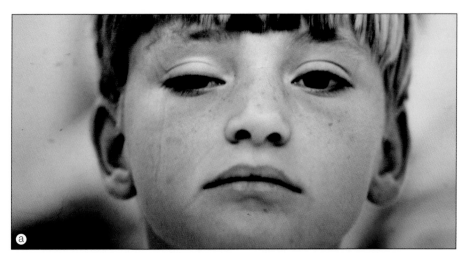

Figure 12.5 (a) Marcus Gunn jaw winking ptosis.

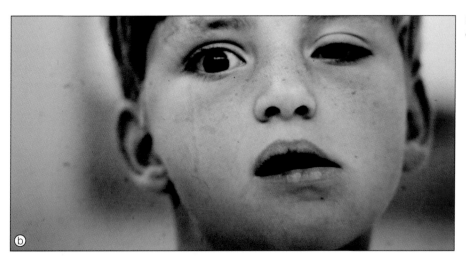

Figure 12.5 (b) When the jaw is moved to the opposite side, the ptosis is relieved.

Blepharophimosis is typically an autosomal dominant trait and includes the findings of congenital ptosis, telecanthus, epicanthus inversus, phimosis, and lateral displacement of the inferior punctum. For patients with significant telecanthus, ptosis repair usually follows repair of the telecanthus by way of transnasal wiring. This is then followed by frontalis suspension.

Patients with myasthenia gravis are thought to have an immunological blockage at the level of the neuromuscular junction, resulting in an effective lack of acetylcholine. The ptosis is often severe, with poor levator function. Diplopia may be present. The evaluation consists of appropriate diagnostic assays for neuroreceptor blocking antibodies, the Tensilon (edrophonium chloride) test and muscle biopsy, followed by therapeutic use of systemic medications (Mestinon) to see if the ptosis can be improved. Significant ptosis that is functionally disabling can be treated with frontalis suspension utilizing an adjustable 1mm silastic rod. It has been reported in the literature that approximately 5–10% of myasthenia patients have Graves' disease. Ptosis may occur in hyperthyroidism and therefore patients with Graves' disease who manifest ptosis with poor levator function should be screened for myasthenia gravis.

Chronic progressive external ophthalmoplegia may have a myogenic as well as neurogenic origin. The patient may present with bilateral, severe ptosis and absence of extraocular movements to a varying degree in each eye, but typically does not report diplopia. The pupillary reflexes are typically normal. The levator function is poor. Some of these patients may have associated involvement of the periorbital orbicularis muscles, and some even have paresis of the frontalis muscles of the forehead. Since these patients have absent Bell's protective eye movement due to their absent extraocular movement, with a poor orbicularis function causing poor eyelid closure, treatment of ptosis is best managed using an adjustable technique like the frontalis suspension with a 1mm silastic rod.

Among the neurogenic ptosis category, one would include Horner's syndrome as well as third nerve palsy. Horner's syndrome can occur with involvement of the primary, secondary, or tertiary fibers of the sympathetic nervous system. The most often mentioned causes include tumors (e.g. Pancoast tumor of the lung), trauma, aneurysms, and iatrogenically from surgery. The manifestation includes mild ptosis with excellent levator function, relative miosis of the pupil, anhidrosis, and a greater degree of anisocoria in dark as compared with light setting. Third nerve palsy may occur with diabetes, orbital trauma, tumors, vascular episodes, infections, as well as neurologic emergencies. The manifestation includes severe ptosis with poor levator function and paralysis of the superior rectus, inferior rectus, medial rectus, and inferior oblique. The ptotic upper lid when lifted shows an eye in a downward and out-turned position, due to the remaining actions of the lateral rectus and the superior oblique muscles. Cases that do not resolve after at least 6 months may be treated with strabismus correction followed by ptosis repair in the form of adjustable frontalis suspension, preferably using a 1mm silastic rod.

Mechanical ptosis, as the name implies, may include aging-related dermatochalasis, fatty prolapse, presence of abnormal tissues (hemangiomas), tumors as in plexiform neuroma of Von Recklinghausen's syndrome (neurofibromatosis), and patients with floppy eyelid syndrome (pachydermoperiostosis – constellation of sebaceous hyerplasia, recurrent blepharitis, and meibomitis; thickened, engorged, and elastic upper tarsi, and spontaneous out-turning of the tarsal plates, especially during sleep). Mechanically, scar bands may occur following surgery, trauma, or idiopathic conditions like ocular pemphigoid and Stevens–Johnson syndrome. Cicatricial reaction along the skin as well as within the middle lamella (orbicularis, orbital septum, preaponeurotic fat, levator muscle) can cause a mechanical tethering of the levator muscle, resulting in ptosis.

EVALUATION AND TREATMENT

Clinically, the patient's past history as well as findings would help one determine whether the patient has congenital versus acquired ptosis. Evaluation should include the following assessments, in rough order of clinical significance:

1. levator function;
2. amount of actual ptosis and functional impairment;
3. presence or absence of protective eye mechanism;
4. tear functions;
5. absence or presence of lid crease; and
6. age of patient – especially in the pediatric age group.

Levator function (LF), in general, guides the surgeon into the following paths:

■ LF = 0–5mm – frontalis suspension procedure;

■ LF = 6–10mm – external levator resection; and

■ LF = 11mm or above – Fasanella–Servat procedure, tarso-aponeurotic resection of McCord, aponeurotic repair/tuck/advancement/ resection, and internal müllerectomy.

To document the amount of ptosis, the normal upper lid margin should cover the upper end of the cornea by 1.0 to 1.5mm. In elderly patients, this normal may be set at 2mm below the corneal limbus. If an adult's upper lid position covers 5mm of his or her cornea on one eye and the other side is normally situated at 1.5mm, the difference or net amount to be corrected will be 3.5mm. (That is assuming the patient is orthophoric; if the patient is not orthophoric, strabismus surgery ought to be considered first, to correct for any vertical deviation.) Documentation of functional impairment should be carried out on each ptosis patient using visual field evaluation and photography, for medico-legal as well as insurance accountability purposes.

Absence of Bell's phenomenon and tear function anomaly should prompt one to be more conservative in the overall degree of surgical repair. If a patient has poor extraocular muscle movement (as in chronic progressive external ophthalmoplegia), despite a moderate levator function (LF = 5–10mm), the patient should not have any levator or aponeurotic resection. Instead, he or she should have an adjustable frontalis suspension.

In the pediatric age group, a ptotic young child without significant threat of amblyopia ought to be conservatively managed until the age of 4 or 5 years, at which time the measurements are more accurate and the anesthetic risk for the child is reduced.

The presence of a lid crease in a ptotic child with a history of relatively normal lids at birth and onset of ptosis later on in life should indicate a need for a lesser degree of resection of levator muscle. Conversely, a congenitally ptotic child with good levator function (LF >11mm) will still need a greater degree of aponeurotic and/or levator muscle resection than his or her normal adult counterpart, as the child's levator muscle is dystrophic and less responsive to each millimeter of resection.

Surgical Repair

For the majority of cases of acquired ptosis seen in an ophthalmologist's practice, with LF ≥11mm

External tarso-aponeurotic resection (of McCord)

The upper lid is anesthetized from the conjunctival side superior to the tarsus as well as from the skin side. The tarsus is everted and the height of the tarsus measured; this helps in placement of the lid crease incision (the lid crease will be the lower line of incision if some redundant skin–orbicularis is to be excised). The skin is incised with a No. 15 Bard-Parker type blade. The orbicularis along the superior tarsal border is traversed horizontally to expose the anterior tarsal surface as well as the distal insertion of the levator aponeurosis. McCord originally determined the amount of resection by adding 3mm to the amount of ptosis to be corrected. For example, if one needs to lift the lid 3.5mm, the amount to be resected will be 6.5mm (3.5 + 3.0). It is then marked out over the plane of the tarsus and aponeurosis, such that half of the 6.5mm is on the aponeurosis side and the rest is over the tarsal plate.

After making sure that a corneal protective shield is in place, resection is carried out by first incising through the tarsal plate with a No. 15 blade and then cutting out the spindle-shaped segment of tarsus and aponeurosis with sharp spring scissors. Bleeding will be at both corners of the wound from the superior tarsal arterioles and may be easily controlled with bipolar wetfield cautery. A double-armed 7-0 silk suture is used to take an anterior tarsal bite along the central portion of the superior cut edge of the tarsus (aligned at or just nasal to the pupillary center), then each of the suture ends are passed through the cut superior edge of the levator aponeurosis. Two additional double-armed sutures are similarly placed, one medially and one laterally along the superior tarsal border. The three sutures are temporarily tied and the contour adjusted to effect an ideal lid shape. The sutures are then permanently tied. The lid crease wound may be closed with a 7-0 silk suture, or enhanced by concurrent placement of five to six 6-0 silk sutures in a skin–aponeurosis–skin fashion.

Advantages

McCord's technique allows for accurate placement and design of the lid crease, removal of skin–muscle redundancy in an elderly patient, an open view, assessment of integrity of the levator muscle, more accurate contouring of the palpebral fissure in case of dehiscence of the medial horn of the levator, and avoidance of lateral peaking, as well as medial undercorrection of the ptosis that may often be seen with Fasanella–Servat correction, which is a posterior approach tarso-Müller-aponeurectomy. It may require a greater degree of familiarity with eyelid anatomy.

Chen's modification – modified external tarso-aponeurectomy of McCord

This is a very useful technique that may easily be performed in conjunction with an upper blepharoplasty. The upper lid is anesthetized from the conjunctival side superior to the tarsus as well as from the skin side. The tarsus is everted and the height of the tarsus measured; this helps in placement of the lid crease incision. The skin is incised in a full-thickness fashion with a No. 15 blade or needle tip of a radiofrequency unit. The orbicularis over the superior tarsal border is then traversed horizontally to expose the anterior tarsal surface as well as the insertion of the levator aponeurosis. The amount of resection is determined by adding 2mm to the actual millimeters of ptosis to be corrected. For example, if one needs to lift the lid 2.5mm, the amount to be resected will be 4.5mm (2.5 + 2.0). It is then marked out over the plane of the tarsus and aponeurosis, such that 1–2mm of it is over the tarsus and the rest is over the aponeurosis (**Fig. 12.6**).

After making sure that the corneal protective shield is in place, resection is carried out by first incising through the tarsal plate with a No. 15 blade and then cutting out the spindle-shaped segment of tarsus and aponeurosis with a pair of sharp spring scissors (Wescott) (**Fig. 12.7**). Bleeding will start at both corners of the wound from the superior tarsal arterioles and may be easily controlled with bipolar wetfield cautery or radiofrequency unit.

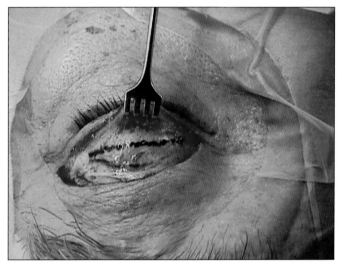

Figure 12.6 Modified tarso-aponeurectomy: the amount of tissue to be resected is marked unequally across the tarso-aponeurotic junction.

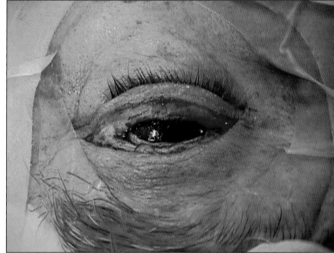

Figure 12.7 The tarso-aponeurotic tissue has been excised in a full-thickness segment, exposing the black eye protective scleral shell beneath.

A double-armed 7-0 silk suture is used to take an anterior tarsal bite along the central portion of the cut edge of the tarsus (aligned at or just nasal to the pupillary center), then each of the suture ends are passed through the superior cut edge of the levator aponeurosis. Two additional double-armed sutures are similarly placed, one medially (over the medial one-third) and one laterally (over the lateral one-third) along the superior tarsal border (**Fig. 12.8**).

The suture placement may be adjusted up or down, or loosened before being permanently tied (**Fig. 12.9**). The lid crease wound may be closed using a 7-0 silk suture; alternatively, it may be enhanced by concurrent placement of five to six 6-0 silk sutures in a skin–aponeurosis–skin fashion, or reinforced using three separate transcutaneous pretarsal fixation sutures from the aponeurosis to the pretarsal inferior skin edge.

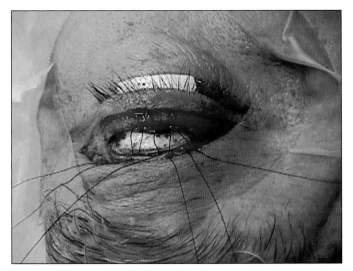

Figure 12.8 Three double-armed 7-0 black sutures have been placed from the anterior surface of the superior edge of the tarsus to the levator aponeurosis.

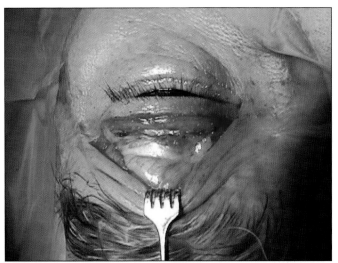

Figure 12.9 The sutures have been tied and the levator aponeurotic complex (with Müller's muscle and conjunctiva) is firmly attached to the tarsus, without any exposed suture knot that may irritate the underlying cornea.

Discussion

McCord originally proposed the use of an 'add-on' factor of 3mm to be added to the amount of desired lift; and it was originally designed to lift the upper lid margin to a point 1mm below the superior corneal limbus. I have been setting the ideal level now in elderly patient to 2mm below the limbus, i.e. 1mm lower than I used to, and therefore I currently use 2mm as the add-on factor in determining the amount of tarso-aponeurectomy.

The original method described distribution of the resection equally over the tarsal plate and the levator aponeurosis. I have not had to straddle equally over the superior tarsus and then resect more than 1–2mm of the tarsus plus levator aponeurosis since most patients exhibit ptosis no worse than around mid-pupil or half of their cornea (where 5mm of the cornea is covered by the upper lid). In this situation with 5mm of cornea being covered, to lift the eyelid to a point 2mm below the superior limbus, the lift factor is 3mm (5 – 2), plus the add-on factor of 2mm, resulting in 5mm of resection. I would then choose to include 1.0–1.5mm of tarsus and 3.5–4.0mm of the distal levator aponeurosis for resection. The resected specimen includes Müller's muscle, levator aponeurosis, as well as conjunctiva. In patients whose ptosis covers more than half of the cornea, resection using the above formula while resecting no greater than 2mm of the tarsus seems to yield equally satisfactory correction (**Fig. 12.10**).

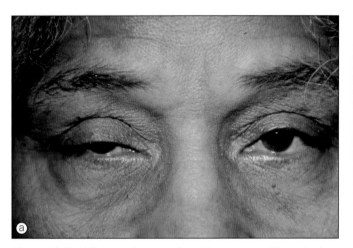

Figure 12.10 (a) Preoperative view of an elderly woman with acquired aponeurotic ptosis. Note the higher right upper lid crease.

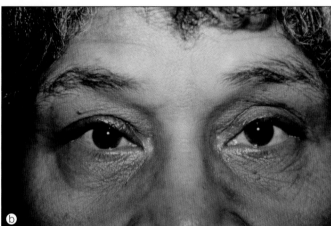

Figure 12.10 (b) Postoperative view after tarso-aponeurectomy.

The effective lift from resection of these tissues is just as effective, millimeter for millimeter, as when actual tarsal plate is being resected (**Fig. 12.11**). To preserve as much of the upper tarsus as feasible, the doctrine of resecting no more than 2mm of tarsus seems to yield as good a result as equal straddling of the superior tarsal border as long as the appropriate amount of aponeurosis is resected in an atraumatic fashion. It is quite possible that when correcting a greater degree of ptosis by this modified tarso-aponeurectomy, one is farther from the superior tarsal border and is resecting levator aponeurosis that is not as thinned out or degenerated. It may also arise because elderly patients have a weaker opposing preseptal orbicularis oculi muscle (which is an antago-

nist to levator and an agonist for eyelid closure), resulting in an equally effective ptosis repair when some skin, preseptal orbicularis, and aponeurosis are resected in combination with very minimal tarsal resection. The atraumatic fashion with which a surgeon can handle the resection and the inherent skill improvement with repetition no doubt add to the predictability of this procedure.

Individual ocular and orbital factors, as well as the relative position of the opposite eyelid of the patient, will necessarily determine the adjustments that works well with one's surgical technique. This modification preserves a major portion of the tarsus, and the ptosis repair may be repeated as necessary in future should the ptosis continue to recur with advancing age.

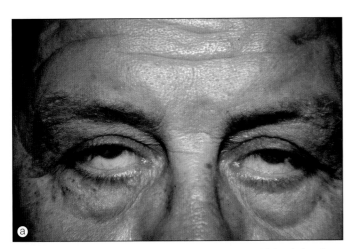

Figure 12.11 (a) Preoperative view of an elderly man with involutional ptosis.

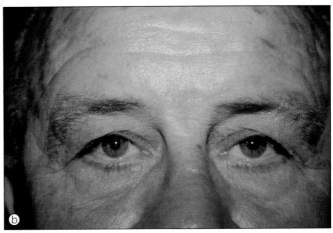

Figure 12.11 (b) Postoperative view after external tarso-aponeurectomy.

Aponeurotic repair/aponeurotic tuck/aponeurotic advancement/aponeurotic resection

These are essentially variations of exploration of the levator aponeurosis via the anterior skin approach. There are situations when the dehisced edge of the levator aponeurosis is clearly detectable on exploration and reapproximating it in a graded fashion on the antero-superior border of the tarsal plate may correct the ptosis. Some surgeons use a single 6-0 or 7-0 silk suture; others use two or three 6-0 Vicryl sutures for this purpose. More often though, there is true stretching, rarefaction, and secondary lengthening of the aponeurosis, and therefore a resection of at least twice the amount of the ptosis to be corrected, combined with reattachment, is necessary. Again, the reattachment may be performed using three double-armed 7-0 silk sutures as described in the section on external tarso-aponeurectomy.

Fasanella–Servat procedure for correction of minimal ptosis (posterior approach, from conjunctival side)

This used to be a popular and often taught method for correction of simple acquired ptosis, mild to moderate in measurement, with LF greater than 11mm.

The upper lid is anesthetized from the conjunctival side superior to the tarsus as well as from the skin side. A corneal protective shell is applied. The upper lid is everted and two curved hemostats are used to clamp symmetrically onto a segment of the tarsus, equal to the amount of ptosis to be corrected. It is important to place the two instruments such that they are evenly applied on the medial as well as the lateral portion of the upper tarsus, that they meet in the center and the midpoint is aligned with the physiologic pupillary axis. One must also be aware of any lateral migration of the tarsal plate (easily detected when the upper lid is everted) (Fig. 12.3), a finding often confirmed intraoperatively in elderly patients who may have dehiscence or fatty degeneration of the medial portion of the levator (medial horn of the levator) (Fig. 12.2). The tips of the hemostat clamps should be angled closer to the lid margin near the central portion of the lid, to avoid the common problem of central peaking. 6-0 plain catgut sutures are passed in a continuous mattress fashion from the lateral end to the medial end just above the clamps. The tissues circumscribed by the clamps (tarsus, Müller's muscle, and some strands of levator aponeurosis, as well as conjunctiva) are then resected using a No. 15 blade. The clamps are then removed and the catgut sutures are externalized onto the skin side through the cut edge along the superior tarsal border. They are adjusted to ensure a good lid contour and correction of the ptosis, and are then tied.

Müllerectomy (posterior approach, from conjunctival side)

For the patient who has 1–4mm of ptosis, good levator function, and a positive response to 2.5% or 10% phenylephrine (lessening of ptosis after instillation of this drop), this is a viable alternative. It involves resection of the Müller's muscle from a posterior conjunctival approach and is therefore less apt to be used in conjunction with a cosmetic blepharoplasty. (Interested readers may refer to Putterman's original paper, listed in the Further Reading section.)

For patients with LF 5–10mm: levator resection

Patients with fair levator function often will benefit from an external resection of the levator muscle. The lid is approached through a lid crease incision. The surgeon traverses through the preseptal orbicularis in a beveled fashion until the orbital septum is reached. The septum is opened horizontally across the width of the eyelid fissure with spring scissors. A Desmarres retractor is used to gently hold back the preaponeurotic fat pads. Two small buttonholes are made through the levator–Müller's muscle–conjunctiva, one medially and one laterally, just above the superior tarsal border. A Berke ptosis clamp is applied along the levator aponeurosis's insertion onto the tarsus with the handle pointing towards the lower lid, and the muscle disinserted using a No. 15 blade. (**Fig. 12.12**). The ptosis clamp, with the levator–Müller–conjunctiva in place, is turned over to expose the conjunctival side. A conjunctival incision is made on this side next to the edge of the clamp. The conjunctiva is carefully dissected off as a layer from the overlying Müller's–levator muscles. (Care must be taken to avoid tearing or buttonholing the flap; a helpful maneuver is to infiltrate the conjunctival flap with some saline or lidocaine with 1:100 000 dilution epinephrine.) As the dissection proceeds halfway towards the superior fornix, it is helped by the use of a cotton-tipped applicator. The conjunctival edge is then sutured back onto the superior tarsal border using a 6-0 Vicryl suture. The clamp now has anywhere from 15 to 20mm of levator aponeurosis and levator muscle, as well as Müller's muscle.

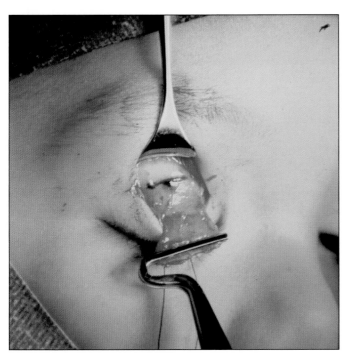

Figure 12.12 External resection of levator muscle of right upper lid. The levator to be resected is held by a Berke ptosis clamp.

Dissection and severance of the medial and lateral extensions of the levator (the 'horns') are to be avoided if possible since it is thought that this lessens the lift per millimeter of levator resected. The appropriate amount of resection is usually between 16 and 18mm, and this is marked on the levator. Three double-armed 6-0 Dexon sutures are placed along the antero-superior edge of the upper tarsus, and then each end is applied through the underside of the levator muscle at the marked sites. The levator muscle is advanced and tied down. The muscle is resected. The ends of the double-armed 6-0 Dexon sutures are then applied along the upper and lower skin edges to facilitate formation or reformation of the lid crease (**Fig. 12.13**). The crease wound is closed with additional 6-0 nylon or absorbable sutures (**Fig. 12.14**).

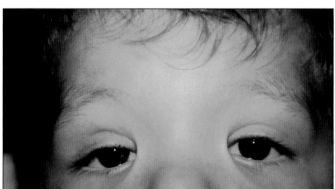

Figure 12.14 Same child as in Figure 12.4, after levator resection.

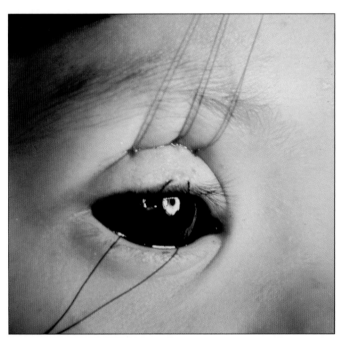

Figure 12.13 Three double-armed 6-0 Dexon sutures function as a crease-forming suture.

Empirical tables correlating desired upper lid margin position intraoperatively to preoperative levator function are often used. An example of such is shown in **Table 12.1**.

Patients should be counseled preoperatively that lagophthalmos may likely occur or be worsened following surgery. Artificial tears and ocular lubricant nightly are helpful adjuncts. The upper lid usually relaxes after 4–5 months and the globe will then be adequately protected as long as there is a good Bell's eye protective mechanism (**Fig. 12.15**).

The exception to use of this technique for patients with moderate levator function of 5–10mm would be patients with Marcus Gunn jaw winking ptosis. These patients are better managed with extirpation of their aberrant levator muscle, coupled with bilateral frontalis suspension.

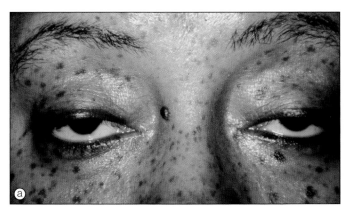 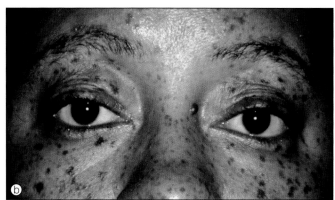

Figure 12.15 Adult woman (a) before and (b) after levator resection.

Table 12.1: Levator resection for patients with levator function 5–10mm (under general anesthesia).	
Levator function	Desired intraoperative lid margin
5–6mm	Place it 1.0–1.5mm above desired level
7–8mm	Place it at desired level plane
9–10mm	Place it 1mm below desired level

For patients with LF of 0–5mm: Frontalis Suspension

For those with poor levator function, the classical frontalis supension is really the only available option, assuming that the patient has a functioning frontalis muscle. Problems postoperatively include undercorrection, corneal exposure, lid margin contour abnormality, asymmetry, and lagophthalmos. It is not a very satisfactory solution and in some segments of the oculoplastic community, it is not enthusiastically endorsed.

Adjustable frontalis suspension using a 1mm silastic rod

Indications include patients with myogenic ptosis (myotrophic dystrophy, myasthenia gravis, chronic progressive external ophthalmoplegia; congenital ptosis where the patient is too young to yield sufficient autogenous fascia lata) as well as neurogenic ptosis (Marcus Gunn ptosis).

Under general anesthesia, the surgeon applies a corneal protective shield over each eye. A No. 15 blade is used to make a 10mm skin incision over the central portion of the eyebrow, just above the hairline. Three small subcutaneous incisions (3mm each) are made over the pretarsal region of the upper lid, just below the lid crease or superior tarsal border, medially, laterally, and centrally. A Keith needle may be bent into a gentle curve and then passed from the supra-brow incision, staying between the periorbital orbicularis and the underlying levator muscle, to exit through the small infra-crease incision medially. A length of 1mm silastic rod is threaded through the eye of the Keith needle and retrieved back towards the supra-brow incision. A straight Keith needle is used to thread the 1mm silastic rod horizontally across the tarsus in an epitarsal manner. In this maneuver, exiting through the central infra-crease incision and then repassing it and the 1mm silastic rod to the lateral infra-crease incision makes the passage more controlled.*

7-0 silk is used to tie down the silastic rod along each of the three infra-crease incisions, taking an intratarsal bite, before any attempt is made to lift the lid with the 1mm rod. The original curved Keith needle is then repassed through the brow incision, exiting through the lateral infra-crease incision to redirect the silastic rod back towards the brow incision. Over the supra-brow incision, a silastic Watzke sleeve (retinal buckling synthetic element) is expanded with a micro-hemostat and each end of the silastic loop is passed through the sleeve, allowing the sling to be tied down and adjusted to the proper tension. Again, empirical tables are used, an example of which is shown in **Table 12.2**.

---

*Clinical point: If a patient does not have a crease, the tarsus is everted and the distance from the central lid margin to the superior tarsal border is measured with a caliper; this is where a physiologic upper crease ought to be placed on the skin side. Full-thickness lid-crease-forming sutures like Pang's sutures are seldom necessary, as the sling will crease a fold over the superior tarsal border, mimicking an upper lid crease, providing the pretarsal portion of the synthetic sling is adequately fixated.

Table 12.2: Frontalis suspension for patients with levator function 5–10mm (under general anesthesia).	
Levator function	**Desired intraoperative lid margin**
0–2mm	Place it 1mm above desired level
3–4mm	Place it at desired level plane
5mm	Place it 1mm below desired level

The two ends of the silastic rod within the Watzke sleeve are further tied on the outside with a 4-0 Polydek suture (ME-2 needle, by Deknatel), and then it is secured to the upper cut edge of the deep frontalis muscle. Upward movement of the frontalis will pull the upper lid margin via the action of the sling. It is important to check for this, even though the patient is in a supine position, to make sure that the lid margin's elevation is physiologic and not lifted away from the surface of the globe. The brow incision is closed in the deep layer with a 4-0 Vicryl suture and on the skin side with a 5-0 nylon suture, in an interlocking stitch. Each of the three infra-crease skin incisions is closed with a single 6-0 absorbable stitch.

Advantages and disadvantages The use of 1mm silastic rod instead of autogenous fascia lata allows for subsequent access to the tract of the sling and readjustment of the lid position, should there be need for tightening (to reverse undercorrection) or loosening (to reverse overcorrection). This is especially advantageous for patients who have neurogenic or myogenic ptosis, where postoperative results are often unpredictable. It also obviates the need for harvesting the patient's own fascia lata.

There is a higher incidence of undercorrection or loss of the sling's effectiveness with time. Infection has been reported, although this is easily managed with antibiotics, and, when necessary, the silastic rod can be easily removed.

Frontalis suspension using autogenous fascia lata

For adolescents and adults who have congenital ptosis with poor levator function in the absence of other neurologic or muscular conditions, one may elect to harvest fascia lata from the lateral thigh of the patient. A Crawford fascial stripper is used to harvest a 10cm × 10mm band of fascia in a young child, or a 15cm × 10mm band in an adult. The 10mm gives enough width to then subdivide the band into four strips, each 2.5mm wide. This is sufficient for those surgeons who prefer to suspend the lid by two triangles on each side rather than through a single, trapezoidal sling. The fascial strip is tunneled across the lid and along the anterior tarsal surface using a pediatric Crawford fascia needle.

The steps involved in the passage of these fascial strips are as listed in the previous section on frontalis suspension using a silastic rod. After the lid level has been adjusted appropriately, the fascia lata strip is tied at each end. The fascial knot is re-enforced with a 4-0 Polydek suture and then anchored to the underlying frontalis muscle on the upper edge of the suprabrow incision. It is important not to anchor it to the underlying cranial periosteum as this will result in an immobile eyebrow.

FURTHER READING

Anderson RL. Aponeurotic ptosis surgery. Arch Ophthalmol 1979;97:1123–8.

Bedrossian EH. HIV and banked fascia lata. Ophthal Plast Reconstr Surg 1991;7:284–8.

Callahan M, Beard C. Ptosis, 4th edn. Birmingham: Aesculapius; 1990.

Collin JR, Beard C, Wood I. Experimental and clinical data on the insertion of the levator palpebrae superioris muscle. Am J Ophthalmol 1978;85:792–801.

Crawford JS. Repair of ptosis using frontalis muscle and fascia lata. Trans Am Acad Ophthalmol Otolaryngol 1956;60:672–8.

Crawford JS. Repair of ptosis using frontalis muscle and fascia lata: a 20-year review. Ophthalmic Surg 1977;8:31–40.

Dresner SC. Further modification of the Mueller's muscle-conjunctival resection procedure for blepharoptosis. Ophthal Plast Reconstr Surg 1991;7:114–22.

Fasanella RM, Servat J. Levator resection for minimal ptosis: another simplified operation. Arch Ophthalmol 1961;65:493–496.

Frueh BR. The mechanistic classification of ptosis. Ophthalmology 1980;87:1019–21.

Jones LT, Quickert MH, Wobig JL. The cure of ptosis by aponeurotic repair. Arch Ophthalmol 1975;93:629–34.

Linberg JV, Vasquez RJ, Chao GM. Aponeurotic ptosis repair under local anesthesia. Prediction of results from operative lid height. Ophthalmology 1988;95:1046–52.

McCord CD Jr. Eyelid surgery: principles and techniques. Philadelphia: Lippincott-Raven; 1995.

Older JJ, Dunne PB. Silicone slings for the correction of ptosis associated with progressive external ophthalmoplegia. Ophthalmic Surg 1984;15:379–81.

Pang HG. Surgical formation of upper lid fold. Arch Ophthalmol 1961;65:783–4.

Putterman AM, Urist MJ. Mueller muscle-conjunctiva resection. Arch Ophthalmol 1975;93:619–23.

Schechter RJ. Ptosis with contralateral lid retraction due to excessive innervation of the levator palpebrae superioris. Ann Ophthalmol 1978;10:1324–8.

Shore JW, McCord CD. Anatomic changes in involutional blepharoptosis. Am J Ophthalmol 1984;98:21–7.

Tillett CW, Tillett GM. Silicone sling in the correction of ptosis. Am J Ophthalmol 1966;62:521–3.

Wagner RS, Mauriello JA Jr, Nelson LB, Calhoun JH, Flanagan JC, Harley RD. Treatment of congenital ptosis with frontalis suspension: a comparison of suspensory materials. Ophthalmology 1984;91:245–8.

Botox

Jemshed A Khan

Chapter 13

Introduction and History

One of the safest, simplest, and most satisfying methods of elective cosmetic reduction of facial rhytids is by the injection of botulinum neurotoxin type A (BoNT-A, Botox). BoNT is currently injected into selected superficial musculo-aponeurotic system (SMAS)-type facial muscles to temporarily reduce associated static and dynamic wrinkles. BoNT-A relaxes muscles by preventing the presynaptic release of the neurotransmitter acetylcholine at the peripheral cholinergic motor neuron endplate (**Fig. 13.1a & b**).

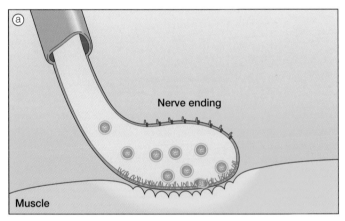

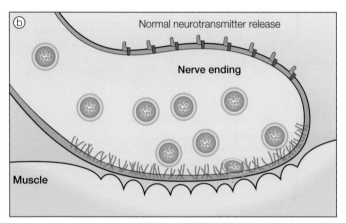

Figure 13.1 (a) Normal skeletal muscle contraction results when there is presynaptic release of the neurotransmitter acetylcholine (ACh) at the peripheral cholinergic motor neuron endplate or nerve ending. The ACh molecules diffuse across the synapse in order to stimulate skeletal muscle contraction.

Figure 13.1 (b) ACh is stored in vesicles residing in the motor nerve ending. Docking of ACh-containing vesicles with the nerve membrane is a necessary step prior to release of the neurotransmitter into the neuromuscular junction. Docking is mediated by a number of molecules including SNAP-25A (blue). ((Courtesy of Allergan Inc.) (Continued overleaf)

Acetylcholine is stored in vesicles residing in the motor nerve ending. Docking is a necessary step prior to release of acetylcholine into the neuromuscular junction. BoNT-A prevents the docking and exocytosis of these acetylcholine vesicles to the nerve endplate. In order for BoNT-A to exert this effect, it must first be absorbed into the nerve ending by a process termed receptor-mediated endocytosis. After BoNT-A is internalized within a cytoplasmic vesicle, the light chain is released into the cytoplasm. The light chain cleaves a protein known as SNAP-25A, which must be functional in order for acetylcholine vesicles to dock prior to release into the neuromuscular junction (**Fig. 13.1c–f**).

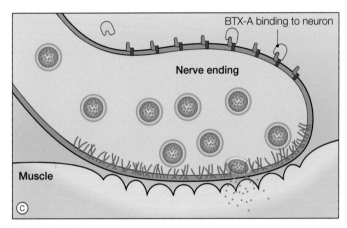

Figure 13.1 (Continued) (c) Following botulinum neurotoxin type A (BoNT-A) injection, molecules of BoNT-A (yellow and gold colored molecules) diffuse through the tissues and bind to the surface of the nerve ending via specific surface receptors (red and blue structures).

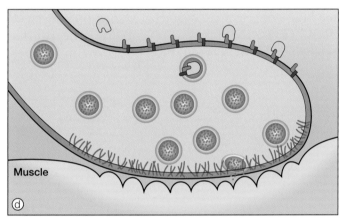

Figure 13.1 (d) After BoNT-A molecules bind to nerve endings, they are absorbed into the nerve ending through a process termed 'receptor-mediated endocytosis'. BoNT-A is then internalized into cytoplasmic vesicles.

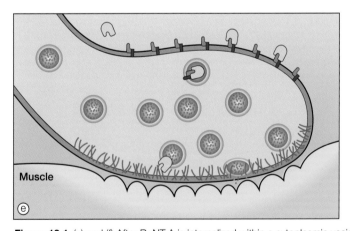

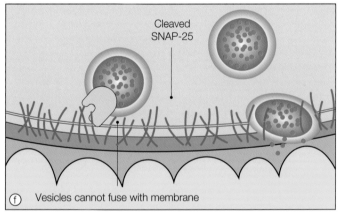

Figure 13.1 (e) and (f) After BoNT-A is internalized within a cytoplasmic vesicle, the light chain of the molecule (yellow) is released into the cytoplasm. The light chain cleaves a protein known as SNAP-25A (blue), which must be functional in order for Ach vesicles to dock prior to release into the neuromuscular junction.

Several distinct immunological BoNT serotypes exist (A, B, C1, D, E, F, G), which vary from approximately 300kD to 900kD. All BoNT serotypes target one or more specific intracellular proteins necessary for synaptic release of neurotransmitter. Proteins targeted by different serotypes include SNAP-25, syntaxin, and vesicle-associated membrane protein (VAMP, also known as synaptobrevin). Over time, the nerve ending may sprout additional axons, which establish new motor endplates (**Fig. 13.1g**). This results in a gradual return of motor function. Skin testing for allergy to BoNT-A is not necessary, although blocking antibodies may occur in patients who receive high doses repeatedly.

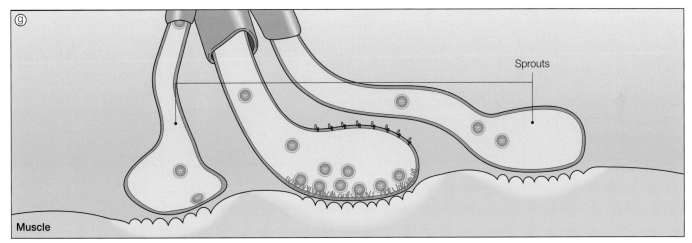

Figure 13.1 (g) The muscle inactivity produced by BoNT-A injections is temporary because peripheral nerve ending sprouts eventually develop and re-innervate the skeletal muscle. (Courtesy of Allergan Inc.)

History of botulinum toxin

- In 1895, Emile Pierre van Ermengem, of Belgium, identified *Bacillus botulinus*

- In the 1920s, botulinum toxin type A was isolated in purified form by Herman Sommer at the University of California, San Francisco, USA

- In 1946, Edward J Schantz and colleagues purified botulinum toxin type A in crystalline form

- In the 1960s and 1970s, Alan B Scott tested botulinum toxin type A in monkeys to determine if the drug might be an effective therapy for strabismus

- In 1978, Dr Scott received permission from the Food and Drug Administration (FDA) to test botulinum toxin type A in human volunteers

Anatomy

The facial mimetic muscles are specialized for several functions, including facial signaling and communication. Most of the muscles of facial expression are part of a continuous interconnected layer of muscle and connective tissue known as the SMAS layer (**Fig. 13.2**). While these muscles are specialized for facial expression, there is also a decline with age in the accuracy with which these muscles convey facial expression. Hence, the age-related development of standing glabellar furrows may create a mistaken expression of disapproval. It is often the goal of Botox injection to reduce the facial 'miscues' through selective pharmacologic denervation of the offending muscles. The common target muscles are summarized in **Table 13.1**.

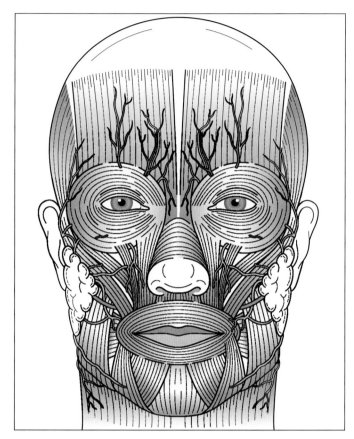

Figure 13.2 Muscles of facial expression.

Table 13.1: Target muscles for botulinum neurotoxin injection.		
Muscle	Action	Primary effect and wrinkle(s) produced when untreated
Orbicularis oculi (orbital portion)	Forced eyelid closure, lateral eyebrow depression	Crow's-feet, eyebrow depression
Corrugator supercilii	Depresses and adducts medial half of eyebrow	Glabellar frown lines
Procerus	Depresses medial eyebrow	Horizontal nasal bridge lines
Depressor supercilii	Depresses head of eyebrow	Depresses head of eyebrow
Frontalis (occipitofrontalis)	Furrows forehead, elevates eyebrows	Horizontal forehead lines
Orbicularis oris	Purses and puckers lips	Vertical lip lines
Depressors of mouth: depressor labii inferioris, depressor anguli oris	Depress lateral angle of mouth	Ptosis of lateral commissure
Platysma	Maintains smooth neck skin	Vertical neck bands

Clinical Indications and Patient Selection

Botulinum neurotoxin type A injection works well and reliably in the crow's-feet, glabella, and forehead (**Fig. 13.3**). With experience, the eyebrows may be repositioned through treatment of the adjacent orbicularis oculi, procerus, corrugator supercilii, and depressor supercilii. BoNT-A may also be used with caution and experience to reduce the perioral rhytids and to improve the lateral angle of the mouth. However, the risk of perioral treatment resides in the possibility of inducing a neurolytic incompetence of the oral sphinter, which may result in temporary drooling or inability to whistle. BoNT-A is not helpful in the treatment of the nasolabial and marionette lines because such treatment results in facial ptosis. Dose is often individualized and may be related to muscle mass, such that relatively smaller doses are sometimes used in females and Asians (**Table 13.3**).

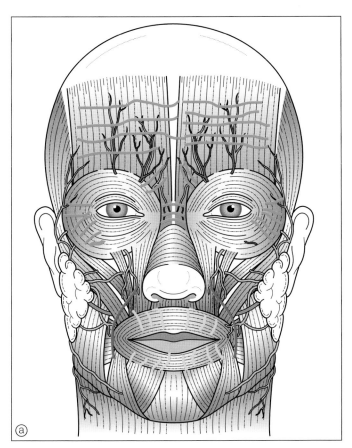

Figure 13.3 (a) Wrinkles indicated for Botox treatment: green wrinkles respond well; yellow wrinkles should be treated cautiously; red lines should not be treated.

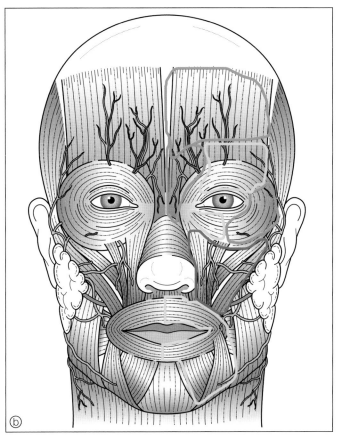

Figure 13.3 (b) Facial zones and underlying muscle groups. Green areas respond predictably and well. Caution is used in yellow areas because of unwanted effects such as adynamic and ptotic eyebrow. Red areas will produce unwanted effects such as drooping cheek and mouth.

Table 13.2: Glogau wrinkle classification scale.

Type I	No wrinkles
Type II	Wrinkles in motion
Type III	Wrinkles at rest
Type IV	Only wrinkles

Table 13.3: General guidelines for typical botulinum neurotoxin type A cosmetic doses.

Site	Dose per site	Number of injections per side	Total dose per side	Spacing of ipsilateral injection	Recommended initial dose per side/ # injection sites per side/ distance between injections
Forehead	2.5–5u	2–5	10–15u	1–3cm	2.5u/2/3cm
Glabella	5–10u	1–2	10–20u	1–2cm	5u/2/1+cm
Crow's-feet	3–10u	1–5	10–15u	1–2.5cm	5u/2/1+cm
Upper lip	1–1.5u	1–2	1–2u	1.5cm	1u/1/na
Lower lip	1–1.5u	1–2	1–2u	1.5cm	1u/1/na
Lateral commissure	5–10u	1–2	5–10u	1–1.5cm	5u/1/na
Platysma	5u	Variable	15–50+	1–3cm	5u/variable/1.5+cm

na, not applicable.

Preparation

Botulinum neurotoxin type A is an extremely labile lyophilized albumin and neurotoxin cryoprecipitate that must be reconstituted without agitation so as to prevent inactivation of effect. Preserved or preservative-free saline is used for reconstitution The author uses 2.2mL of saline as diluent because approximately 0.1mL remains in the vial through capillary attraction to the glass surface (**Fig. 13.4, Table 13.4**).

The reconstituted drug should be used within 4 hours according to the manufacturer's recommendation. A fine 27- or 30-gauge needle is used for administration. Significant residual volume of drug may be wasted in the hub of a detachable 27- or 30-gauge needle: the author prefers the economy of an insulin syringe with a permanently attached needle.

The saline diluent should be dripped into the vial slowly so as to avoid creating a streaming jet of fluid that may agitate and inactivate the labile toxin.

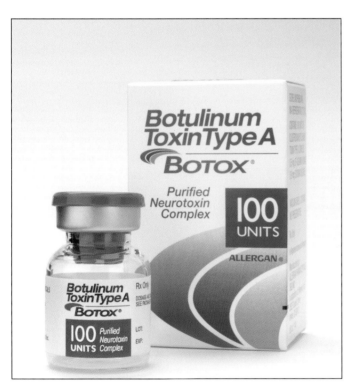

Figure 13.4 Vacuum-sealed vial + 2.2mL saline = approx. 5u/0.1mL.

Table 13.4: Effect of diluent volume on final concentration.		
Saline diluent	Concentration per 0.1 mL	Concentration per 1.0 mL
1.0mL	10u	100u
2.0mL	5u	50u
2.5mL	4u	40u
4.0mL	2.5u	25u
10mL	1.0u	10u

Preparation

1. Store in freezer prior to use

2. (Optional step) Break seal and remove stopper

3. Drip in saline slowly, 2.2mL

4. 2.2mL non-preserved saline = approx. 5u/0.1mL

5. Roll gently to mix – do not shake or stir

6. Withdraw 0.5 or 1.0mL via insulin syringe without dulling tip

7. Refrigerate unused portion and use within 4 hours

Injection Techniques

General principles

The purpose of injection is deliver an appropriate intramuscular or perimuscular drug dose while minimizing the risks of bruising and pain. Because of the thinness of the overlying skin, ecchymosis is easily visible when it arises from the orbicularis oculi muscle. Thus, it is better to inject subcutaneously over the orbicularis oculi muscle and thereby avoid direct intramuscular injection and visible ecchymosis. Ecchymosis may also result from transection of fine subcutaneous vessels; therefore, it is important to look for and avoid such vessels when injecting in the crow's-feet area. Superficial injection may be delivered by perpendicular or tangential placement of subdermal BoNT-A to relax the frontalis muscle. Application of pressure immediately and directly to the injection site will minimize bruising. In the areas of thicker dermis overlying the orbicularis oris, mouth depressors, and corrugator supercilii muscles, one may attempt intramuscular injection since the thick overlying tissue will obscure ecchymosis.

Gently pinching the skin overlying the procerus, corrugator, and frontalis muscles may help reduce discomfort and ensure superficial placement of drug (**Fig. 13.5**). One may also reduce discomfort with topical anesthesia techniques including ice, EMLA, Betacaine LA, etc.

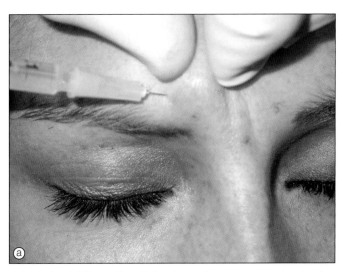

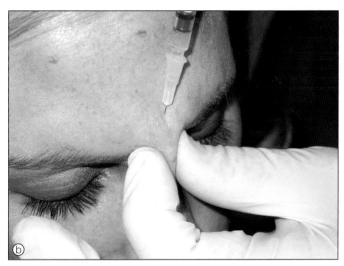

Figure 13.5 (a) The pinch technique is used to ensure correct anatomic placement of the needle tip over the corrugator supercilii and to reduce discomfort.

Figure 13.5 (b) A similar technique is employed to treat the procerus muscle. (Courtesy of Rick Anderson, MD.)

Crow's-feet injection

Crow's-feet injection is one of the simplest and most satisfying applications of BoNT-A. The radiating dermal crow's-feet lines result from the concentric constriction of the underlying orbital and preseptal orbicularis oculi muscle (**Fig. 13.6**). The orbicularis oculi injections of BoNT-A may result in diminution of both active and static crow's-feet rhytids, may prophylactically delay the onset and progression of such wrinkles, and improves final outcome following laser ablative periocular resurfacing. The thin periocular skin is prone to visible bruising; therefore, injection should be delivered in the subdermal plane while avoiding actual intramuscular injection. The loose periocular subdermal plane in the area of crow's-feet rhytids should visibly balloon up when the injection is delivered at the proper depth. Following injection, the patient may apply pressure with facial tissues for 1–2 minutes over the injection sites, to minimize bruising.

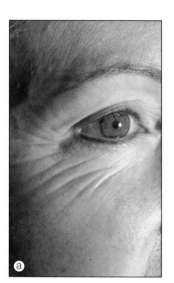 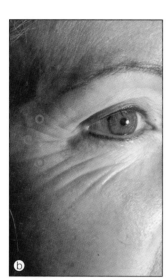 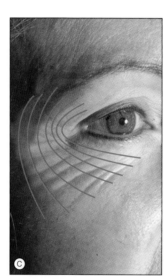 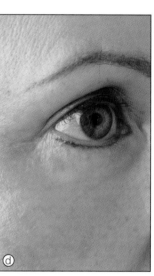

Figure 13.6 (a) Crow's-feet rhytids. (b) Typical injection sites for radiating crow's-feet rhytids. (c) Location of underlying concentric orbicularis oculi muscle fibers. (d) Improvement in rhytids following botulinum neurotoxin type A injection. (Courtesy of Joan Kaestner, MD.)

Essentials

- Consciously avoid visible vessels
- Insulin syringe with integrated 30-gauge needle
- Injection sites 1–2cm lateral to lateral canthal angle
- 10–15u total dose per side, divided into two to five injections per side
- Injections 1–5cm apart
- Apply pressure after each injection

Corrugator and Procerus Rhytid Treatment

Cosmetic injection of Botox for glabellar rhytids was approved by the FDA in April 2002 (**Fig. 13.7**). To reduce pain and avoid blunting the needle tip during injection, care should be taken, respectively, to avoid injecting too shallow or too deep: stay deep enough to be subdermal, but not so deep as to engage the periosteum. Pain may also be reduced by palpating the supraorbital notch and thereby avoiding the vertical course of the supraorbital nerve. Stay 0.5cm superior to the eyebrow to reduce the risk of eyelid ptosis.

The procerus muscle may be injected in the midline or by pinching the nasal bridge and entering the procerus tangentially. The drug is deposited in the midline. Generally, a single procerus injection is placed over the upper nasal bridge either at or up to 7mm higher than the level of the medial canthal tendon.

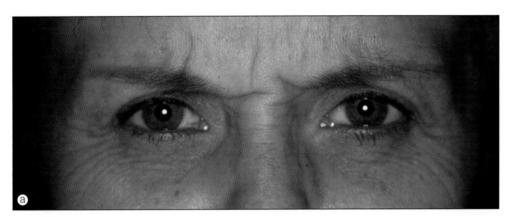

Figure 13.7 (a) Glabellar and horizontal procerus wrinkles.

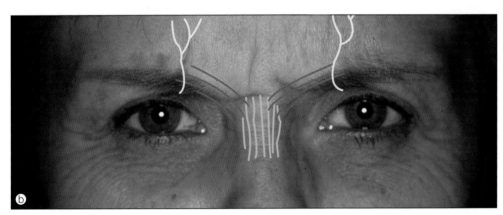

Figure 13.7 (b) The corrugator muscles are represented by red lines. The procerus muscle location is depicted by green lines. Note the course of the supraorbital nerve (yellow) located 2.5cm lateral to the midline and often also located by palpating the supraorbital notch. The inferior portion of the nerve should be avoided because of pain or ecchymosis due to injection of the nerve or laceration of the accompanying blood vessels

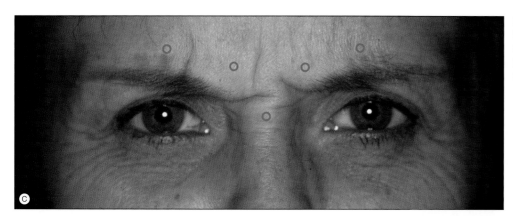

Figure 13.7 (c) Typical injection sites. Five injection sites of 5u each are typically used. Note that the lateral site is never placed directly superior to the supraorbital notch.

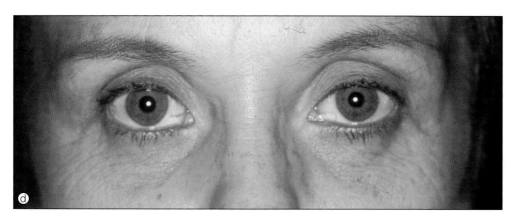

Figure 13.7 (d) Improvement in rhytids following botulinum neurotoxin type A injection. Note the smoother appearance to the glabellar area. (Courtesy of Joan Kaestner, MD.)

Essentials of treatment for glabellar rhytids

- Perpendicular or tangential injections
- Insulin syringe with integrated 30-gauge needle
- Avoid supraorbital neurovascular bundles
- Avoid dulling the needle against the periosteum
- Inject at subdermal or intramuscular depth
- Deeper depth is more painful
- Injection sites placed at least 0.5cm superior to the upper eyebrow border
- Injection sites placed at least 0.5cm medial or lateral to the path of the supraorbital nerve
- Two injections of 5u each delivered to each corrugator muscle and 5u into the procerus
- Apply pressure after each injection

Essentials of treatment for procerus

- Procerus muscle is midline structure
- Procerus action creates horizontal furrows
- Emotional signal created by procerus action is aggression
- Inject 5u into the midline procerus

Frontalis Treatment

Frontalis injection is useful in treating horizontal forehead wrinkles. Injection sites are at least 1–2cm above the eyebrows to avoid a ptotic or adynamic and expressionless eyebrow. Injection should be delivered across the medial and lateral frontalis to avoid segmental eyebrow elevation (see complications section of this chapter). A series of two injections per ipsilateral forehead is usually a good starting point, and may be increased to ten sites, depending upon patient response (**Fig. 13.8**).

Prior to injection, one should search for any underlying eyelid ptosis with compensatory eyebrow elevation. Forehead injection and the resulting eyebrow depression may worsen an underlying eyelid ptosis in such patients.

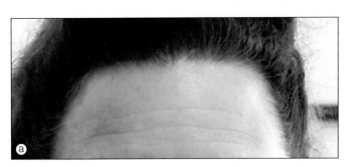

Figure 13.8 (a) Note horizontal forehead furrows prior to injection.

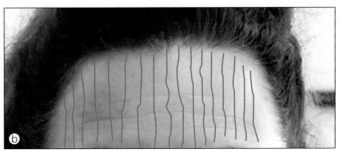

Figure 13.8 (b) Red lines depict the location of the vertically oriented frontalis muscle.

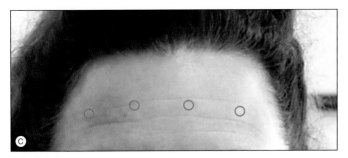

Figure 13.8 (c) Four injection sites of 1.5–4.0u per site is a safe beginning dose.

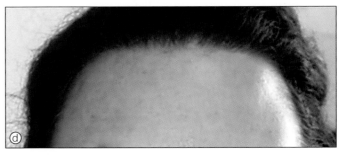

Figure 13.8 (d) Smooth forehead appearance 2 weeks following injection.

Essentials

- Frontalis is a paired muscle, connected to the posteriorly located occipitalis muscle

- Frontalis action raises the eyebrows and furrows the forehead

- The emotional signal created by frontalis action is surprise

- Usual injection dose is 1.5–4.0u per site

- Usually, there are between four and ten injections sites per patient, depending upon the size of the forehead

- Use proper technique to avoid brow ptosis

- Use proper technique to avoid adynamic eyebrows

Advanced Techniques: Perioral

The perioral area responds less predictably than other treatment areas because the dynamic muscle actions associated with eating, drinking, speaking, and smiling may be impaired. Therefore, a cautious approach to this area is warranted (**Figs 13.9 & 13.10**).

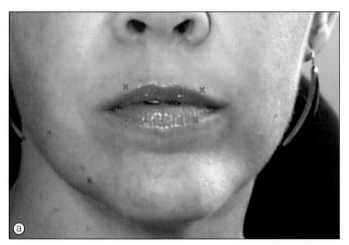

Figure 13.9 (a) Typical treatment sites for vertical lip lines. Minute doses, i.e. 1.0–1.5u per site, are delivered. The dose and number of injection sites may be gradually increased if the response is inadequate. Only 50% of patients are satisfied with perioral Botox because of drooling, difficulty puckering and whistling, and impaired enunciation.

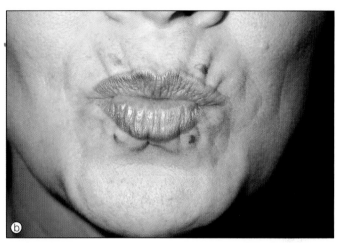

Figure 13.9 (b) Patient with vertical lip lines demonstrating ability to pucker prior to injection. (Courtesy of Rick Anderson, MD.)

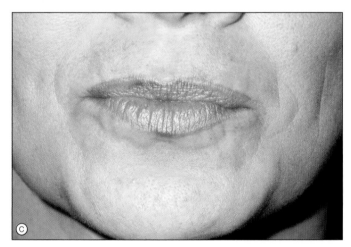

Figure 13.9 (c) Same patient following Botox injection demonstrates inability to pucker despite voluntary effort. (Courtesy of Rick Anderson, MD.)

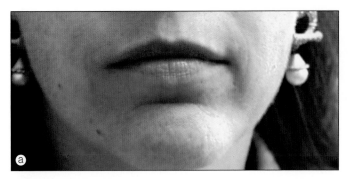

Figure 13.10 (a) Preoperative appearance of patient with depressed lateral oral commissures. Note the slight downward angulation of the lateral oral commissures prior to injection.

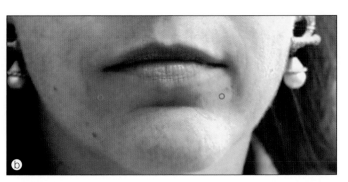

Figure 13.10 (b) Injection sites for treatment of depressed lateral oral commissures. Generally, 5–10u per site is delivered.

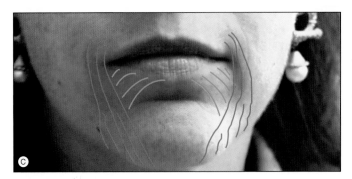

Figure 13.10 (c) Overlay of perioral muscles. Red lines represent depressor anguli oris. Green lines represent depressor labii inferioris. Both muscles may be targeted for Botox treatment.

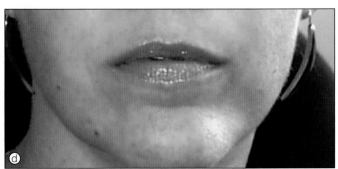

Figure 13.10 (d) Note subtle improvement in wrinkles and slight elevation of the lateral oral commissures 2 weeks following injection.

Pitfalls

Only 50% of patients are happy with perioral injections

Complications

Complications may be minimized with appropriate refinement and adjustment of injection sites and doses on subsequent visits. For example, the patient pictured in **Figure 13.11** received supplemental injections to the lateral frontalis muscle to correct the excess temporal eyebrow elevation **Figure 13.12** shows secondary ptosis following BoNT-A.

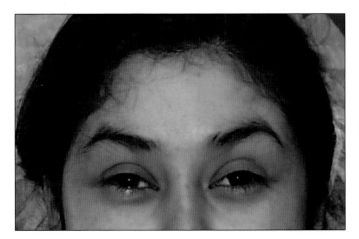

Figure 13.11 Patient complained of temporal eyebrow tenting following forehead botulinum neurotoxin type A (BoNT-A) injections. Placement of additional doses of 5u into each lateral frontalis muscle corrected the eyebrow contour deformity.

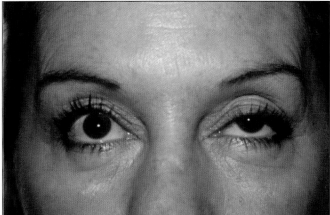

Figure 13.12 Temporary left upper eyelid ptosis following BoNT-A treatment of forehead and glabella.

Essentials

- Complications may be reduced with appropriate dosing

- Complications may be reduced with appropriate anatomic technique

- Ptosis will resolve spontaneously

- Eyelid ptosis may be treated with Iopidine drops or Naphcon-A

- Perioral complications include drooling and inability to whistle

- Diplopia, dry eyes, exposure keratitis, and lagophthalmos are unusual with cosmetic injections

Documentation of Treatment

Anatomic documentation of treatment sites creates a historical record upon which further treatment modifications may be individualized (**Fig. 13.13**). For example, if a patient has inadequate lateral forehead wrinkle reduction, one may refer to the previous treatment diagram and use this as a basis for adding new lateral treatment sites.

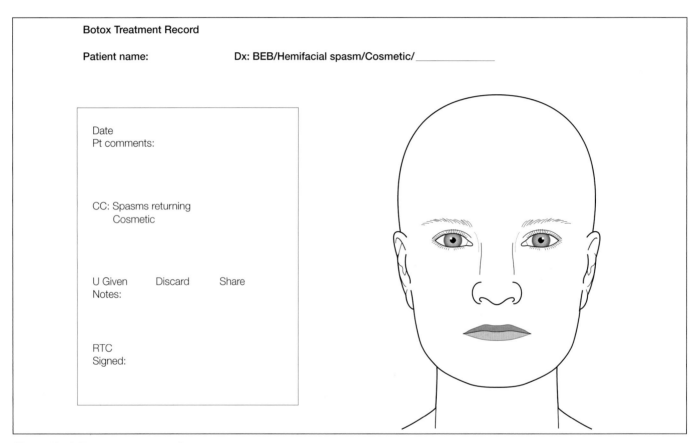

Botox Treatment Record

Patient name: Dx: BEB/Hemifacial spasm/Cosmetic/_____

Date
Pt comments:

CC: Spasms returning
        Cosmetic

U Given   Discard   Share
Notes:

RTC
Signed:

Figure 13.13 Botox treatment record.

Informed Consent

While BoNT-A appears to be a safe and effective drug, the very long-term consequences of neurotoxin injection are unknown. Therefore, informed consent is important despite the relative simplicity of the procedure. Informed consent discussion should refer both to the known side effects as well as to the unknown risks related to the use of human albumin in BoNT-A.

Lifetime Consent for Administration of Botox

1. I, _____ _____
(first name, last name), request that Dr _____, or whomever he designates, administer botulinum toxin to me for either medical or cosmetic purposes. Botox is not FDA approved for headache treatment, tarsorrhaphy, or muscle twitching. Photos of me may be taken and used for educational, scientific, or marketing purposes.

2. If Botulinum is given for medical purposes, such as involuntary muscle spasm, tarsorrhaphy, blepharospasm, hemifacial spasm, muscle twitch or tick, etc, I hereby acknowledge that I understand that there may be alternative treatments for this condition, including, but not limited to, medical therapy including the administration of oral medicines, muscle stripping or other operations, removal of motor nerves, or procedures to release pressure on involved nerves.

3. I acknowledge that I understand that Botox A includes human albumin. Albumin is a protein, similar to the white of a chicken egg, that is derived from human blood products. While it is not believed that there has been any transmission of diseases from Botox A, I understand that this is very unlikely but possible. I accept the risk of the possibility of acquiring an infection, including viral or other types of infections, from Botox administration and accept the risk of unknown future complications from Botox

use. I understand that botulinum B can also be used for my condition and does not contain albumin.

4. Botulinum toxin usually works well in 95% of patients. There is a 5% chance that it will not have an adequate effect. It is not always possible to predict the effect, and it may work too well or not well enough. Some of the side effects may include flu symptoms, headache, temporary droopiness of one or both eyelids or double vision. Permanent muscle weakness is very unlikely.

5. By signing this document, I agree that it includes all botulinum toxin injections already provided by Dr _____ or whomever he designates, as well as all future Botox treatments.

6. I understand that the effects of botulinum toxin use with pregnancy or breast-feeding are not known and that I should not take Botox if the possibility of pregnancy or nursing exists.

7. In summary, the risks, consequences, benefits, and alternatives of treatment, including no treatment, have been explained to me.

Signed (Patient) _____
Date __/__/__

Witnessed By _____
Date __/__/__

Ablative Laser Skin Resurfacing

Jemshed A Khan

Chapter 14

Introduction

Erbium:YAG and CO_2 laser resurfacing systems create a controlled-depth cutaneous ablation and an associated thermal injury zone which is followed by a healing response that produces the desired improvement. In order to ablate skin without scarring, the laser must remove the epidermis and some papillary dermis while minimizing thermal injury. Since the 'chromophore' for the 10.6μm CO_2 and 2.94μm erbium:YAG laser is water, ablation occurs when the laser pulse is sufficient to almost instantaneously raise the intracellular epidermal fluid to its boiling point, at which time a steam plume is ejected out of the wound, quickly carrying away with it the generated heat before significant collateral tissue damage can occur. Subsequent passes with the CO_2 laser must induce thermal, conformational, and other changes in the dermal collagen to induce shrinkage and wrinkle reduction (**Figs 14.1 & 14.2**). Because these thermal effects are thought to prolong healing times, the erbium:YAG lasers are marketed as an alternative 'cool' method of epidermal ablation and wrinkle improvement.

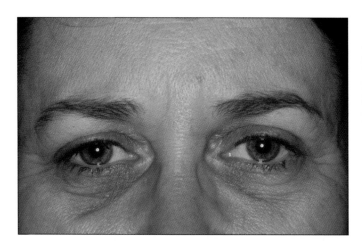

Figure 14.1 Patient prior to periocular CO_2 laser skin resurfacing.

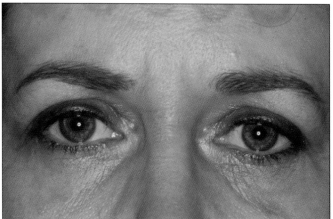

Figure 14.2 Patient subsequent to periocular CO_2 laser skin resurfacing.

Comparison of CO_2 versus Erbium Ablation

Although both CO_2 and erbium wavelengths ablate tissues, more tissue is ablated with CO_2 laser per pulse and the zone of associated thermal injury is greater. The differences between erbium and CO_2 effects are largely related to the longer pulse duration of CO_2 (approximately 1ms) and its greater tissue penetration (**Figs 14.3**).

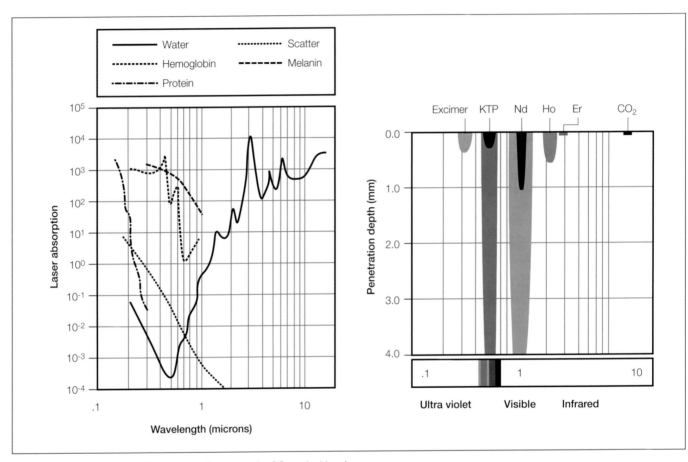

Figure 14.3 Absorption and tissue penetration curves for CO_2 and erbium lasers.

The greater thermal injury and ablation associated with CO$_2$ are advantageous insofar as the patient has a greater improvement in wrinkling and one can resurface further into the vascular dermis without the encumbrance of significant bleeding (**Fig. 14.4**). On the other hand, with erbium one can create a finer degree of epidermal ablation and the patients encounter proportionally quicker recovery times (**Fig. 14.5**). Since erbium wavelength is absorbed more highly by water than is CO$_2$, there is a corresponding difference in the minimal fluences necessary for ablation: for CO$_2$ laser, ablation occurs at or above 4–5J/cm^2, whereas for erbium laser, ablation occurs at 1.6J/cm^2 or higher (**Table 14.1**).

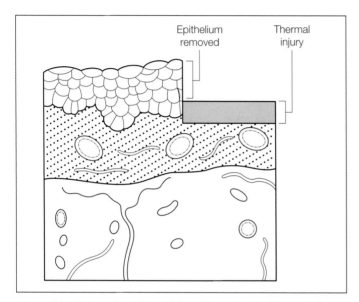

Figure 14.4 Schematic of CO$_2$ ablation. (Reproduced with permission from Khan JA. Laser skin resurfacing. In: Chen WP, ed. Oculoplastic surgery: the essentials. New York: Thieme; 2001:180.)

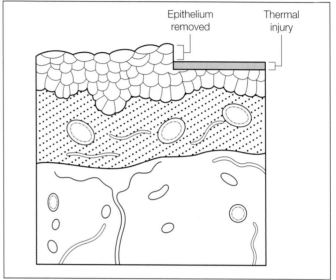

Figure 14.5 Schematic of erbium ablation. (Reproduced with permission from Khan JA. Laser skin resurfacing. In: Chen WP, ed. Oculoplastic surgery: the essentials. New York: Thieme; 2001:180.)

Table 14.1: Comparison of CO$_2$ and erbium lasers.		
	CO$_2$	**Er:YAG**
Ablation fluence	≥4–5J/cm^2	≥1.6J/cm^2
Wavelength	10.6µm	2.94µm
Usual pulse	950µs	250µs
Thermal damage	75–150µm	10–50µm
Vaporization	20–70µm	2–400µm
Tissue penetration	30µm	1µm
Collagen shrinkage	++++	+

Tissue Response

The first CO_2 laser pass vaporizes the epidermis, leaving a residual desiccated debris which is wiped away. By contrast, several passes with the erbium: YAG laser are required to reach equivalent depth. No more resurfacing passes are necessary when the goals of treatment are limited to the epidermis. Subsequent laser passes may be applied to the papillary dermis in order to create deeper ablation. Because of the thermal effects associated with CO_2, there is also an immediately noticeable thermal shrinkage and stimulation of a long-term healing response characterized by deposition of new subepidermal collagen (Grenz zone) and elastin fibers. This tightening of the dermis creates the wrinkle reduction (**Figs 14.6–14.8**).

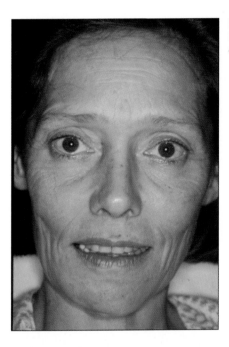

Figure 14.6 Preoperative appearance of age-related facial laxity.

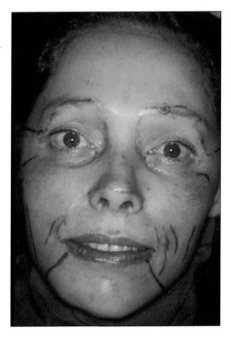

Figure 14.7 Note the improved intraoperative facial appearance resulting from thermal collagen shrinkage and vaporization of the aged epidermis.

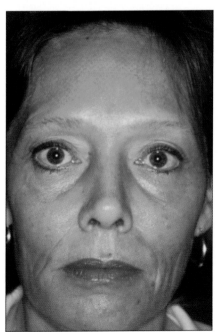

Figure 14.8 Epidermis has healed and regenerated by day 14 with residual erythema.

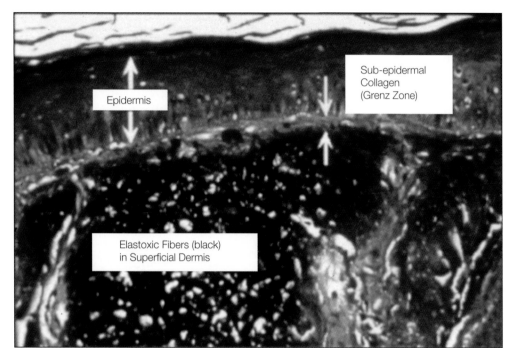

Figure 14.9 Preoperative appearance of thinned Grenz collagenous zone in aged skin. (Image courtesy of Dr Richard Fitzpatrick.)

Epidermis

Sub-epidermal Collagen (Grenz Zone)

Elastoxic Fibers (black) in Superficial Dermis

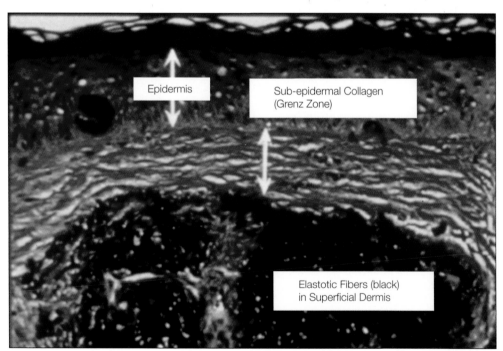

Figure 14.10 Thickened Grenz zone following CO_2 laser skin resurfacing. (Image courtesy of Dr Richard Fitzpatrick.)

Epidermis

Sub-epidermal Collagen (Grenz Zone)

Elastotic Fibers (black) in Superficial Dermis

Wound Healing

Healing after ablative resurfacing requires the re-establishment of the barrier function of the epidermis and appropriate return of normal skin pigmentation. The new epidermis results from the differentiation and surface migration of a reservoir of basal-like keratinocytes residing deep to the epidermis in the pilar complexes. Hence, re-epithelialization may be impaired when the pilar complexes have been inactivated by isoretinoin (Accutane®) use or heavy X-ray irradiation, or destroyed (i.e. very deep resurfacing into the dermis). Hence, caution is prudent, especially when resurfacing the very thin eyelid skin or when attempting to erase very deep wrinkles whose bases may lie at the same depth as the reticular dermis of the adjacent tissue shoulder (**Fig. 14.11, Table 14.2**). Likewise, hypopigmentation may result from deep resurfacing. Scarring may also be more likely in keloid-prone patients or over the edges of facelift flaps. Complete epithelialization is characterized by the cessation of weeping and oozing and a smooth, pink, dry skin surface. In general, re-epithelialization is completed within 7 days for erbium:YAG and 10–14 days for CO_2 resurfacing. Erythema typically takes a few weeks to resolve after erbium:YAG, but lasts around 12 weeks for CO_2 laser.

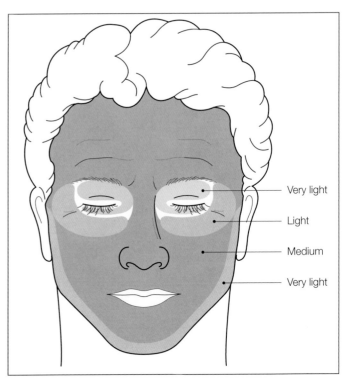

Figure 14.11 Danger zones for resurfacing. Note that the dermis of the neck, mandibular border, and eyelids is especially thin. (Reproduced with permission from Khan JA. Laser skin resurfacing. In: Chen WP, ed. Oculoplastic surgery: the essentials. New York: Thieme; 2001:188.)

Table 14.2: Average thickness of facial skin in microns at various locations.				
Zone Location	**Epidermis**	**Dermis**	**Hypodermis**	**Total**
Neck	115	138	544	797
Eyelids	130	215	248	593
Root of nose	144	324	223	691
Cheek	141	909	459	1509
Lobule of nose	111	918	735	1764
Forehead	202	969	1210	2381
Lower lip	113	973	829	1915
Upper lip	156	1061	931	2148
Mental region	149	1375	1020	2544
Reproduced with permission from Gonzalez-Ulloa M, et al. Preliminary study of the total restoration of the facial skin. Plast Reconstr Surg 1954;13:151–61.				

Preoperative Evaluation

The preoperative evaluation screens for patients who are at a higher risk of complications. Specific features to elicit in the history include immune system compromise and racial origins of African, Far-East Asian, or Native American background. A personal or family history of keloid formation may increase the likelihood of keloid formation or hypertrophic scarring after resurfacing. Fitzpatrick class IV or darker skin is prone to hypertrophic scarring or pigmentary problems (**Table 14.3**). Isoretinoin (Accutane) treatment or past facial X-ray treatments may impair follicle and sweat gland activity, thus resulting in delayed or absent re-epithelialization after resurfacing. Active acne may be accelerated by the intense healing response and trigger further scarring (**Fig. 14.12**). Patients with acne rosacea or telangiectasia may have more noticeable vessels after resurfacing. Lower eyelid laxity may predispose to ectropion (**Table 14.4**).

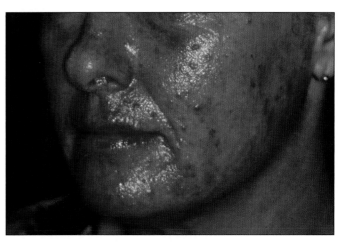

Figure 14.12 Unusually severe acne eruption subsequent to CO_2 laser skin resurfacing. (Courtesy of Bhupie Patel, MD.)

Table 14.3: Fitzpatrick's skin type classification system.		
Type	**Colour**	**Reaction to first sun exposure yearly**
I	White	Always burn/never tan
II	White	Usually burn/tan with difficulty
III	White	Sometimes mild burn/tan average
IV	Medium brown	Rarely burn/tan with ease
V	Dark brown	Rarely burn/tan very easily
VI	Black	Never burn/tan very easily

(Data from Fitzpatrick RE, Goldman MP, Satur NM, Tope WD. Pulsed carbon dioxide laser resurfacing of photoaged facial skin. Arch Dermatol 1996;132: 395–402.)

Table 14.4: Risk factors and relative contraindications to laser skin resurfacing.		
Condition	**Possible outcome**	**Relative risk**
Active acne	Exacerbation, scarring	High
Keloid history	Hypertrophic scarring	High
Fitzpatrick IV–VI skin	Hyperpigmentation	Moderate to high
X-ray facial irradiation	Poor re-epithelialization	Moderate to high
Accutane use in past	Poor re-epithelialization	High
Vitiligo	Dyschromia	High
Phenol peel	Dyschromia	Moderate
Deep dermabrasion	Dyschromia	Moderate
Herpes simplex	Herpetic outbreak	Low with prophylaxis
Immunosuppresion	Infection	Moderate to high
Lower eyelid laxity	Ectropion	Moderate

Prophylaxis

The large raw exposed facial areas following resurfacing may invite devastating bacterial cellulitis (*Staphylococcus aureus*, *Streptococcus pyogenes*, and *Pseudomonas aeruginosa*), primary *Herpes simplex*, or reactivation of latent *Herpes simplex*, with disseminated facial scarring. Therefore, physicians may prescribe prophylactic antibiotic and antiviral medications prior to resurfacing (**Fig. 14.13**), in order to achieve therapeutic levels at the time of treatment (**Table 14.5**). Medications are continued for 12 days thereafter or until re-epithelialization is well established. All resurfacing patients, except those with very small treatment areas, receive a preoperative oral antibiotic, usually ciprofloxacin hydrochloride (Cipro), 500mg orally twice daily for 14 days, beginning 48 hours prior to surgery. Acyclovir (Zovirax), a thymidine kinase inhibitor that is active against human herpes viruses, may be prescribed as 400mg orally every 8 hours for 14 days, commencing at least 2 days prior to surgery.

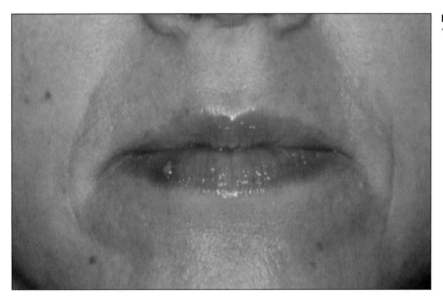

Figure 14.13 Preoperative appearance of herpetic 'cold sore'. Patient procedure was cancelled.

Table 14.5: Resurfacing – prophylactic preoperative care.			
Indication/Class	**Generic name**	**Brand name**	**Recommended**
Antibiotic	Ciprofloxacillin	Cipro	Most cases
Antiviral	Acyclovir	Zovirax	Most cases
Antifungal	Fluconazole	Diflucan	Not recommended
Bleaching agent	Hydroquinone	Various	Fitzpatrick IV–VI
Bleaching agent	Kojic acid	Generic	Fitzpatrick IV–VI
Anticomedogenic	Tretinsin	Retin A	Neutral
Steroid	Hydrocortisone	Various	Use with Retin A
Sunscreen	Various	Various	Neutral

Laser Safety and Anesthesia

Both CO_2 and erbium:YAG wavelengths are invisible to the human eye and hazardous to ocular tissues. Therefore, wavelength-specific protective goggles should be worn by the surgical team, and the patient's eyes should be protected by laser-impenetrable shields (**Fig. 14.14**). In addition, there is a combustion hazard; thus, non-flammable or wet drapes are used. Any tubing carrying oxygen should be non-flammable or wrapped in non-flammable material. The laser plume may contain viral particles: laser safety masks that filter out smaller-sized particles should be worn.

CO_2 and erbium:YAG resurfacing may be performed with topical, local, regional, or general anesthesia. Topical anesthesia alone is generally unreliable and is often supplemented with intravenous or oral administration of analgesics and sedatives. Topical Betacaine seems to provide more effect than EMLA. Local infiltrative anesthesia usually consists of lidocaine with epinephrine. Regional nerve blocks are usually to the supraorbital, supratrochlear, infraorbital, and mental branches of the trigeminal nerve. With general anesthesia or deep intravenous sedation with propofol, local anesthetics are unnecessary.

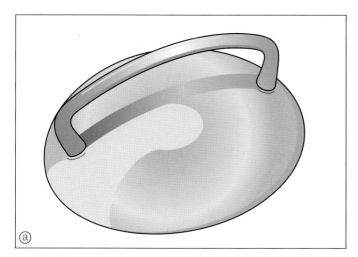

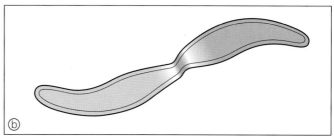

Figure 14.14 (a) A special-finish laser blepharoplasty instrument designed to reduce laser energy reflection: Khan laser eye shield with unique anti-rotational posts and eyelash traction bar for laser-impenetrable globe protection during CO_2 and erbium:YAG laser skin resurfacing. (Source: Bausch and Lomb Surgical/ Storz Instrument Company, St Louis, MO, USA.) (b) Ambidextrous matte-finish titanium Khan–Sutcliffe 'propeller' laser shield used as a backstop during incisional blepharoplasty and to mask off areas during resurfacing. (Source: Bausch and Lomb Surgical/ Storz Instrument Company, St Louis, MO, USA.)

Laser Treatment

CO_2 laser technique:

With CO_2 laser, treatment generally consists of a first pass which addresses epidermal changes by removing the epidermis. The patient is given local anesthetic or topical Betacaine or EMLA cream (**Figs 14.15 & 14.16**).

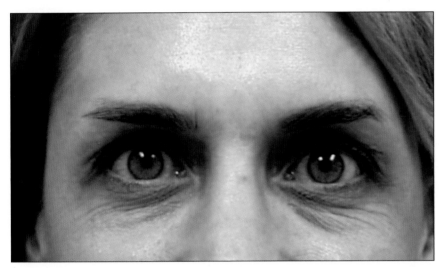

Figure 14.15 Preoperative appearance of periocular rhytids.

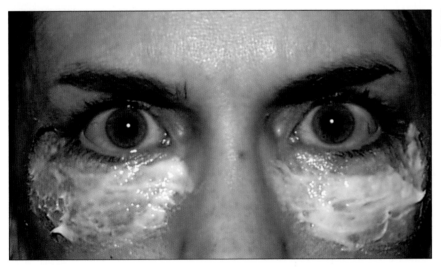

Figure 14.16 The treatment area is outlined with a surgical marking pen, and EMLA cream is applied for topical anesthetic effect.

Debris must be wiped away prior to each subsequent pass, to reduce unwanted thermal injury (**Figs 14.17 & 14.18**). After the first pass, subsequent passes may be applied to the exposed dermis depending upon the severity of wrinkles as well as individual and regional facial tolerances for dermal ablation. Generally speaking, a single pass is applied to the thin eyelid skin, while two or three passes may be tolerated over the crow's-feet, glabella, or upper lip. Only a single pass is prudent as one approaches the thinner skin at the transition from facial to neck skin that occurs over the rim of the mandible. Debris may be left unwiped after the final pass, in order to promote more rapid healing.

Multiple CO_2 laser passes are applied over the thicker skin of the crow's-feet, forehead, glabella, nose, circum-oral areas, and cheeks when the goal is to induce significant dermal remodeling so as to reduce moderate to deep wrinkles. In order to prevent excess thermal damage, debris must be wiped from the dermal surface between passes.

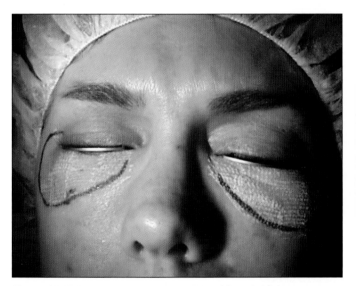

Figure 14.17 White anhydrous carbon-rich epidermal debris corresponding to each individual CO_2 laser spot is evident after the first pass.

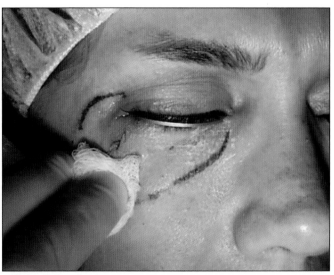

Figure 14.18 The epidermal debris is wiped away prior to subsequent passes in order to avoid a 'heat sink' effect that can create unintended deeper thermal damage. Note the smooth avascular plane of the exposed dermis subsequent to the first pass.

With each subsequent pass, one ablates and induces deeper thermal damage to the dermis. Although this results in greater final wrinkle reduction, one also runs a commensurately increased risk of postoperative scarring, delayed or prolonged healing phase, and dyspigmentation. With each pass, one sees a progressive tightening and yellowing of the dermis (**Figs 14.19 & 14.20**).

There are two endpoints for multiple-pass CO_2 resurfacing. CO2 resurfacing is stopped as soon as any one endpoint is reached. The endpoints consist of either:

1. an arbitrary number of passes (usually one to three passes, depending on the exact area treated); or
2. a smooth and wrinkle-free dermal surface.

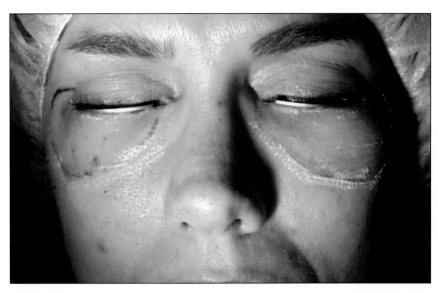

Figure 14.19 Note the scant debris, contracted surface appearance, and slight yellowish coloring ('chamois effect') following the second pass.

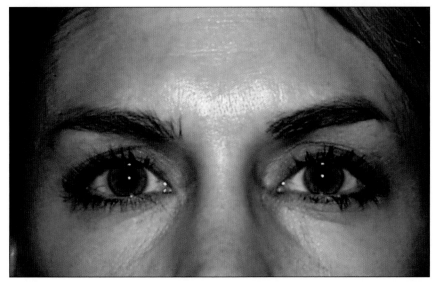

Figure 14.20 Final appearance following CO_2 periocular resurfacing, with marked reduction of rhytids.

Erbium:YAG technique:

With erbium:YAG resurfacing, each pass generally ablates one-fifth to one-third of the epidermis. Therefore, depending upon the depth of treatment, patients may have little or no significant healing time. One may titrate the desired effect from partial to full epidermal ablation and may ablate into the dermis, although this is limited somewhat by bleeding (**Figs 14.21–14.23**).

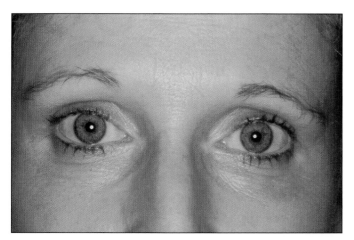

Figure 14.21 Preoperative appearance of mild to moderate periocular rhytids.

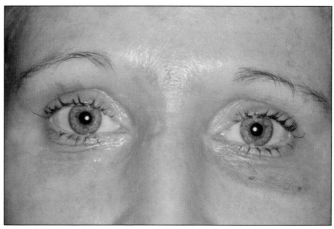

Figure 14.22 Intraoperative appearance following erbium laser treatment of the epidermis. Following three to five passes with erbium:YAG laser, the epidermis has been mostly vaporized. Absence of bleeding indicates that the treatment has not extended significantly into the superficial papillary dermis.

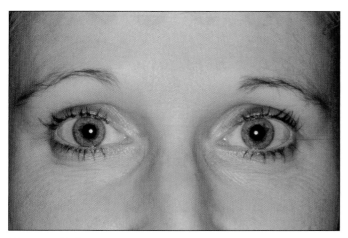

Figure 14.23 Final appearance approximately 2 weeks following erbium:YAG resurfacing. Note the improvement in rhytids and minimal erythema.

Early Postoperative Wound Care

Prior to re-epithelialization, the barrier function of the skin is disturbed and there is leakage and oozing of serum and protein onto the raw dermal surface (**Figs 14.24** & **14.25**). Unsightly crusting, scabbing, and exudate often accumulate on the skin surface. This presents a risk for viral, fungal, or bacterial infection or colonization. Therefore, the goal of postoperative wound care is to promote rapid re-epithelialization. This is accomplished by maintaining a moist surface and avoiding infection.

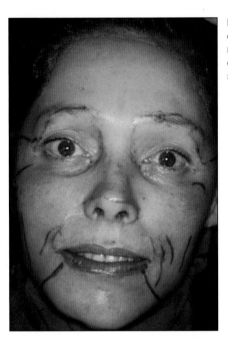

Figure 14.24 At the completion of CO_2 laser resurfacing, the de-epithelialized skin is smooth and moist.

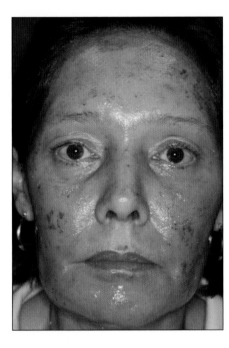

Figure 14.25 By postoperative day 6, the disturbed epidermal barrier allows exudate to dry on the skin surface, resulting in dried debris, crusting, and weeping.

Table 14.6: Products used in immediate postoperative care (prior to complete re-epithelialization).			
Indication/Class	**Generic name**	**Brand name**	**Recommended**
Antibiotic	Ciprofloxacillin	Cipro	Most cases
Antiviral	Acyclovir	Zovirax	Most cases
Antifungal	Fluconazole	Diflucan	As needed
Occlusive dressing	Various	Various	Not recommended
Occlusive topical	Petroleum jelly	Vaseline	Recommended
Occlusive topical	Various	Aquaphor	Recommended
Steroid cream	2.5% hydrocortisone	Various	Recommended
Wound care	Acetic acid	na	Recommended
na, not applicable			

A moist surface is maintained by the application of hydrocortisone cream 1% and Aquaphor four times daily, or application of an occlusive dressing. Occlusive dressings are associated with a higher rate of infection, but benefit the patient in terms of faster re-epithelialization and lessened erythema and postoperative discomfort. Diluted white vinegar and water soaks are applied four times daily, both to loosen exudative crusts and because of their antifungal and antibacterial effects. Oral antibiotics and antiviral agents (and sometimes antifungals) are also helpful. The completion of re-epithelialization is characterized by the appearance of a dry, smooth, pink skin surface (**Fig. 14.26**). Patients should be warned to avoid social and public contact for up to 2 weeks because of the unsightly appearance.

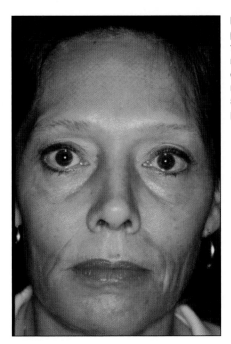

Figure 14.26 By postoperative day 12, the skin has re-epithelialized. The epidermal barrier is re-established, and the skin has a dry, smooth, pink surface.

Late Postoperative Wound Care

Subsequent to re-epithelialization, wound care is designed to hasten the resolution of erythema and minimize postinflammatory hyperpigmentation (**Figs 14.27 & 14.28**). Both conditions are minimized by the topical application of hydrocortisone cream 1% at bedtime for up to 6 weeks after surgery.

Postinflammatory hyperpigmentation is also reduced by the prophylactic use of sunscreen, sun protection factor (SPF) 30 or greater, for 12 weeks after surgery. Topical hydroquinone cream 4% may be applied at bedtime to hasten the resolution of hyperpigmentation (**Figs 14.29 & 14.30, Table 14.7**).

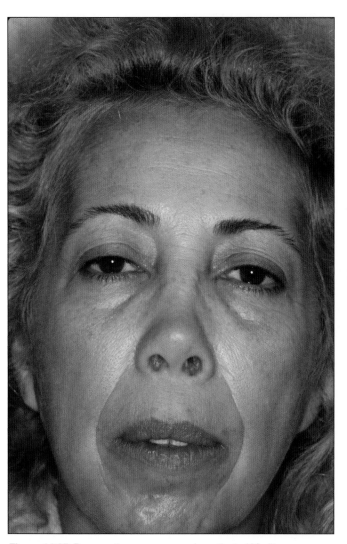

Figure 14.27 Preoperative appearance of a patient of Mediterranean ancestry.

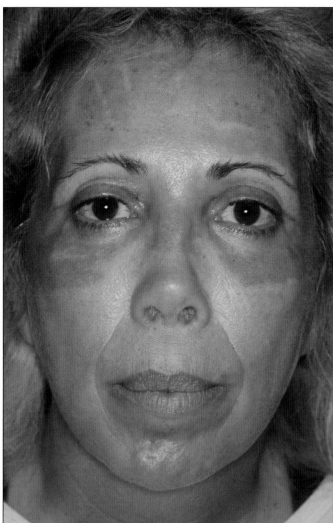

Figure 14.28 Hyperpigmentation present in resurfaced areas about 4–6 weeks after CO_2 laser skin resurfacing.

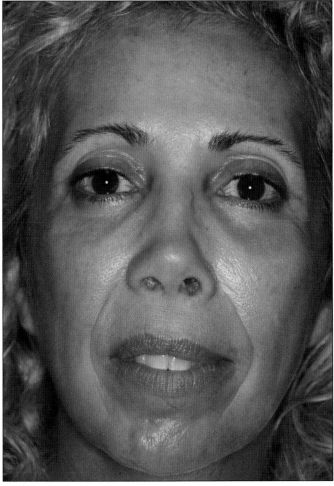

Figure 14.29 Hyperpigmentation has resolved following several weeks' application of topical hydroquinone.

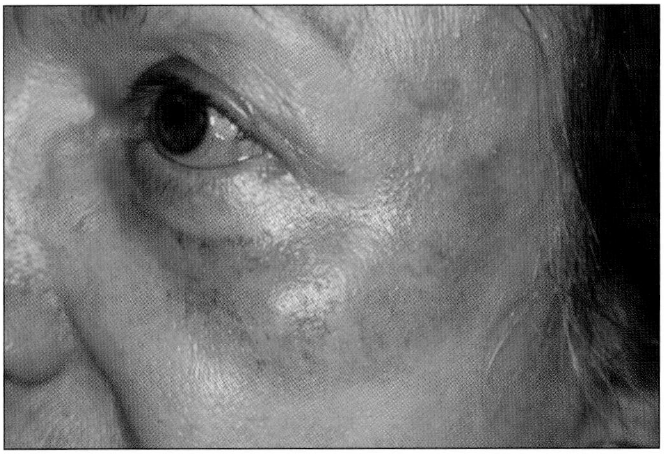

Figure 14.30 Prolonged erythema lasting several months after CO_2 laser skin resurfacing. Erythema resolved with time and topical steroid therapy.

Table 14.7: Products used in late postoperative wound care (after complete re-epithelialization).			
Indication/Class	**Generic name**	**Brand name**	**Recommended**
Steroid cream	Hydrocortisone 2.5%	Various	Recommended
Sunscreen SPF >25	Various	Various	Recommended
Concealer	Various	Various	Recommended
Bleaching agent	Hydroquinone	Various	If pigmenting
Bleaching agent	Kojic acid	Generic	If pigmenting
High-potency steroid	Clobetasol propionate	Temovate-E	If prolonged erythema (Caution: use 1 week only)
SPF, sun protection factor			

Chapter 15

Management of the Eyelid Crease: Advanced Techniques

William PD Chen

The ability to control the location and placement of a crease, as well as the finer quality of a crease, including shape, height, depth, softness, etc., should be a basic skill for any cosmetic facial surgeon. Whether to reset a crease higher or lower, or to create or obliterate a crease, the Asian eyelid surgery model is ideal to study the interplay between the different factors, as the margin or tolerance for errors is quite small. A firm grasp of these concepts will allow one to apply them further onto reconstructive as well as aesthetic cases in all ethnic groups, whether Asians or not. (One can view it in the reverse way – a firm grasp of these factors as practiced in non-Asian patients will allow one to critically apply the skills learnt towards Asian eyelid surgery, where the adverse margin is higher due to the relative lack of redundant skin and intrinsic reactivity of the tissues.)

I will start first by elaborating on some of the parameters controlling an upper lid crease in Asians, then go through some of the suboptimal results encountered, followed by the various surgical solutions. The chapter will conclude with a series of complex revisions to illustrate some of the interplay that goes through my mind as I tackle these cases, in an attempt to lead to an improved outcome and, most of all, a happier patient.

One of the often neglected aspects of preoperative interaction with the patients is a failure to realize that different patients, young or old, whether from Western countries or elsewhere, may have a different concept of what constitutes a beautiful eye accentuated by an aesthetically placed upper lid crease. Some will consider a low-set nasally tapered crease as 'natural' and 'beautiful'. Some like the crease to be shielded somewhat, to give a 'natural look'. Some like a prominent crease, to make the eyelid fissure appear larger, while others like their crease to be relatively shallow or 'soft'. Some want to add constancy to their intermittent and unpredictable crease line; and almost none like it rounded, half-moon shaped, or as high as the supratarsal sulcus. To achieve their chosen aim, patients have been known to try surgeries, and non-invasive means including adhesive eye tapes, surgical glues, and cosmetic glues available in Asia (**Fig.15.1**), or even manual manipulation with various fine tools, sometimes taking 30 minutes to 2 hours every morning.

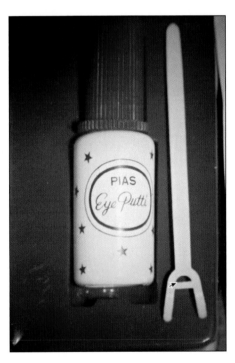

Figure 15.1 One form of glue for non-surgical self-administered formation of eyelid crease: 'Eye Putti' from Japan.

In deciding on the width or height of an Asian crease from the superior lash line, one must be aware that a lower-than-average crease should be no more than 0.5mm (500μm) below that patient's measured tarsal height. Likewise, the upper limit is no more than 0.5mm above the measured height of the upper tarsus, as measured centrally over the middle one-third of the lid margin. Any significant deviation from these values may result in pseudo-ptosis, static crease formation, secondary lagophthalmos, a prominent pretarsal skin zone from chronic edema, and exaggeration of sulcus. The use of buried non-absorbable crease-fixation sutures along the levator aponeurosis over the superior tarsal border may lead to persistent foreign body sensation, upper lid retraction, and scleral show above the superior corneal limbus.

For Asians who request placement of a conservative upper lid crease, removal of preaponeurotic fat is often unnecessary and should be avoided, due to concern that it may lead to a prominent supratarsal sulcus.

Often, physicians are coaxed by the patients into creating a high crease. Asians, in general, have a smaller physique, not only in terms of weight and height but also with respect to the size of their tarsus, their eyelid width, the distance from upper lid margin to the lower border of the brow, etc. Since Western physicians often consider 10–11mm as the average upper eyelid crease height, a crease that they would consider as 'high' will therefore be greater than 9–10mm and much higher than the superior border of the upper tarsus in an Asian. When a 'high crease' as requested by an Asian patient is then constructed by such a physician, it is anatomically inappropriate and aesthetically undesirable, as it tends to lead to lagophthalmos from any placement of 'skin–levator–skin' fixation sutures or 'inferior subcutaneous orbicularis oculi muscle-to-levator aponeurosis' sutures. It is almost always undesirable to create a high crease in Asians: the visual impact is an image of a crease bisecting the zone between the eyebrow and the upper eyelid margin.

Some surgeons advocate that in order to reduce fullness in the pretarsal space, aggressive excision of pretarsal fat and some pretarsal orbicularis oculi should be carried out to ensure that the pretarsal skin lies flat against the tarsus postoperatively. In my practice, I have found that fullness in the pretarsal area is not always undesirable. When the pretarsal area appears expanded and swollen, it is usually the result of a crease that is placed too high to start with, leaving more tissue in between this high crease and the lid margin. Aggressive dissection or excision of pretarsal tissues tends to lead to persistent lymphedema and risks formation of multiple pseudo-creases in the pretarsal region. It is more effective, in my experience, to create a crease fit for that individual that is based on the vertical height of his or her tarsus (measuring 6.5 to 8.0mm), and to excise no more than 2–3mm of the pretarsal orbicularis oculi muscle along the inferior cut edge of the skin incision.

 Clinical pearls

■ Removal of preaponeurotic fat pads in Asian blepharoplasty should be avoided, especially in older patients, to reduce the possibility of enhancing the supratarsal sulcus, a feature that is aesthetically undesirable in Asians.

 Pitfalls

■ It is always undesirable to create a high crease in Asians.

Almost all suboptimal results and complications arise from failure to observe the following points. In patients who do not have a crease and desire Asian blepharoplasty, the only thing that matters to those patients is the new crease line that you will create for them on the upper eyelids. A line can be described by several parameters in mathematics and geometry: it can be described by its *length* (the horizontal extent or width along the superior tarsal border), its geometric configuration (*shape*), its relative separation from the eyelash margin (*height*), and its spatial relationship to the medial and lateral canthi; whether the crease is continuous or broken apart (*continuity*) and whether it stays permanent in appearance (*permanency*) (**Fig. 15.2**). Symmetry between the two lids can occur only if all of the above parameters are accurate, correct, and equally well executed on both sides.

By now one understands that aesthetic Asian eyelid surgery is not as easy as it seems. The surgery demands nothing short of perfection in performing these points. To take the simplest: if the *shape* is not properly chosen (either as a parallel crease or a nasally tapered crease), one can end up with a semilunar crease and a 'westernized' look, which is not what an Asian wants. The Asian patients want to look like their Asian friends who were born with natural, Asian-looking creases. One can also get a bifid crease medially, or one with an exaggerated upward-flare laterally. Asymmetry may occur between the two creases simply because they are different in shape (**Fig. 15.3**).

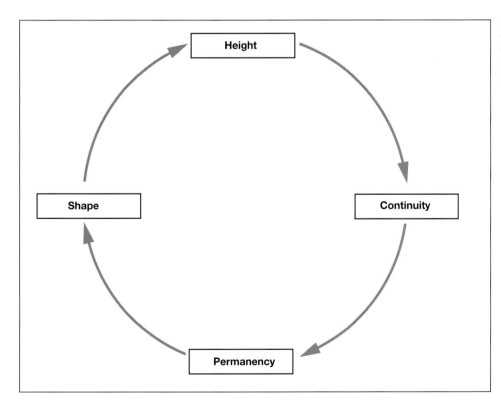

Figure 15.2 Critical parameters for formation of an eyelid crease. (Reproduced with permission from Chen WP. Asian Blepharoplasty: a surgical atlas. Newton: Butterworth–Heinemann; 1995: 56.)

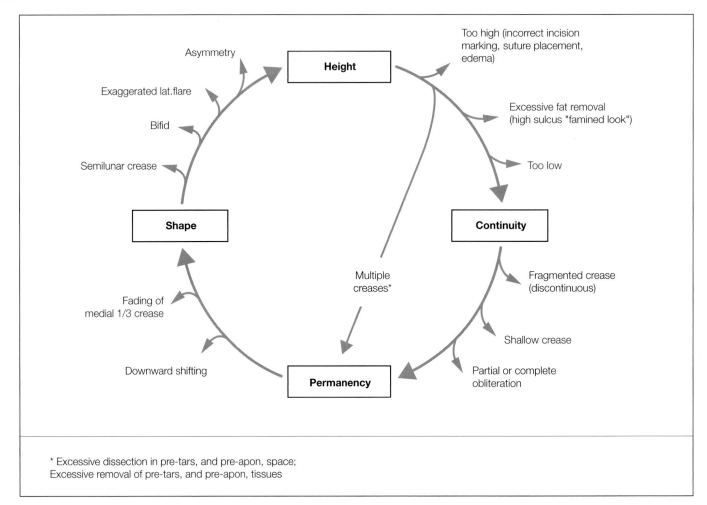

Figure 15.3 Circle of complications in crease formation. Failure to reach each of these parameters or in combination often leads to the findings deviating from this circle of interconnected factors. (Reproduced with permission from Chen WP. Asian Blepharoplasty: a surgical atlas. Newton MA: Butterworth–Heinemann; 1995: 82.)

If the *height* is not properly executed based on the central tarsal height, one can get an excessively high crease (**Fig. 15.4**). It can occur from incorrect placement of the incision line, poor suture placement (onto tarsus, orbital septum, levator aponeurosis, or orbicularis oculi), or persistent edema. A low crease may occur, although it is rare. Excessive fat removal will lead to a 'famined' look with an exaggerated and hollowed supratarsal sulcus (**Fig. 15.5**), which is a suboptimal feature on an Asian face. Multiple creases (**Fig. 15.6**) are more prone to occur if the incision is too high above the superior tarsal border, or if excessive dissection has been carried out along the pretarsal plane or within the preaponeurotic (post-septal) space.

Problems with *continuity* can give rise to a fragmented (discontinuous) crease, a rudimentary shallow but complete crease, or a partially (**Fig. 15.7**) or completely obliterated crease. An otherwise properly formed crease may look obliterated due to inadequate removal of skin and soft tissue above it. This results in hooding of eyelid tissue above the crease, in essence shielding the real crease when the individual is viewed face on, looking straight ahead.

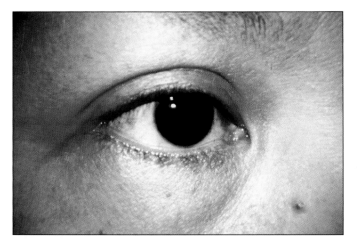

Figure 15.4 A relatively high crease for this Asian lady. Note the dysjunction of the medial end of the right upper lid crease with the medial canthal fold.

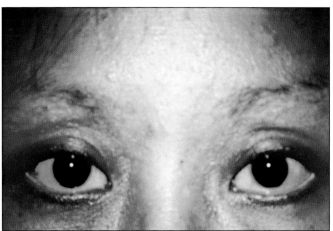

Figure 15.5 Excessive fat removal has resulted in a 'famined' look with a sunken supratarsal sulcus.

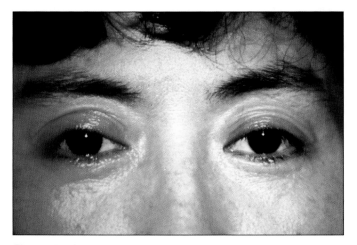

Figure 15.6 Multiple creases are seen over the left upper lid. The right upper lid shows bifid medial crease.

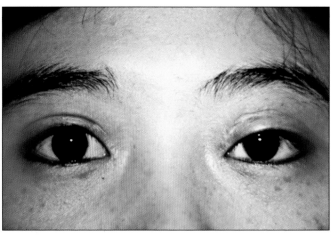

Figure 15.7 The right upper lid has a partial crease as it is incomplete medially. The left crease has disappeared after surgery.

Permanency issues include late disappearance of crease (which is seen more with the conjunctival suturing method widely practiced in Japan and China; **Fig. 15.8**), and downward shifting and progressive shallowing of the crease. The latter arise from inadequate subdermal attachment of the distal fibers of the levator aponeurosis at the level of the superior tarsal border. Fading of the medial one-third of the crease is also a fairly common occurrence and is often due to an inability to adequately fixate the most medial portion of the levator aponeurosis to the skin edges. The result is a crease that is present only over the lateral two-thirds of the palpebral fissure.

If one can achieve correct length (width), correct shape, and correct height, keeping it continuous and permanent, and equally on both sides, then one has eliminated all identifiable surgical inconsistencies and can then hope to achieve symmetry and optimal results – barring unforeseen variables like bleeding (from hypertension, bleeding disorders, and use of herbal medicines and anticoagulants), propensity for scar formation, variation in skin types, and poor patient compliance.

A corollary of this discussion is that any correction of suboptimal results in Asian eyelid surgery requires accurate identification as to which of the above parameters are involved, followed by cooperative blending and reversal of those causes.

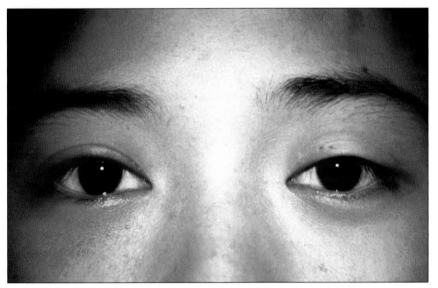

Figure 15.8 Shallowing of crease and complete obliteration and reversion to single eyelid has occurred in this patient's left upper eyelid after suture ligation method.

Revision and Correction of Suboptimal Results

Revision of suboptimal results is a necessary part of any surgeon's repertoire of skills if they are to perform the type of surgery we have been discussing. There are various known factors that will lead to a suboptimal result;[1-7] these include inaccurate placement of crease incision, use of reactive suture materials, excessive bleeding, excessive fat removal, inadequate or excessively tight wound closure, inappropriate techniques, and lack of knowledge on the part of the surgeon.

There are, however, other intangible factors that may be beyond the control of the surgeon – for example, non-compliance to postoperative wound care instructions on the part of the patient; vigorous and immediate postoperative exercises, resulting in prolonged edema of the eyelid margin; latent hypertension with rebleed; unrelated weight gain; unpredictable wound healing in patients who have had multiple revisions before; obsessive patients who are not happy with the results even though the results are fine; or patients who have a preconceived notion of what they expect the crease to do for them (e.g. launch a career in a certain field), even though it may not be attainable.

As previously discussed, the four factors that determine a crease's formation are also the factors that may lead to a suboptimal crease, namely:

- shape;
- height;
- continuity; and
- permanency.

From a patient's perspective, the subjective complaints I encounter most often from patients seeking secondary consultation in my practice are as follows:

1. 'The shape is wrong'.

2. 'The crease is too high' (wrong height).

3. 'My two eyelids are unequal' (asymmetry of crease height on each side, different crease shape on each side, different crease length of each lid [it determines whether the crease looks complete or partial], differences in crease depth [determines the quality or visual softness versus harshness of the eyelid crease]).

4. 'My crease disappeared' (early or late obliteration).

5. 'There is more than one crease' (multiple creases).

6. 'My eyelids look hollowed' (excess fat removal or excessively high anchoring of crease in supertarsal sulcus).

7. 'I want my crease removed!' (rejection of surgically created outcome, wants removal or 'erasure' of crease).

When dealing with the wrong shape, a semi-lunar (half-moon) crease applied onto an Asian eyelid will result in a rounded face (**Fig. 15.9**). For the patient who has a small medial canthal web (medial upper lid fold) and desires a nasally tapered crease, if the medial extent of the crease was not deliberately tailored to merge into and just behind the medial lid fold and it should end up above the fold, one may see a upper bifid crease over the medial end (Fig. 15.4). Rarely, if the medial portion of the crease was overly tapered and went underneath the medial canthal fold, one will see a lower bifid crease. I have seen cases where the lateral portion of a crease was flared up excessively from the lateral canthus, encroaching on the thicker dermis of the eyebrow area.

In terms of height, the crease may be placed too high or too low. Each represents its unique problems. A high crease often looks artificial or surgically created. A low incision may not result in a good crease formation or it may present as an obvious aesthetic blemish over the pretarsal skin platform.

Often seen in conjunction with a high crease is an overzealous removal of the preaponeurotic fat pads. It results in a high supratarsal sulcus or 'famined' look, which is difficult to correct (**Fig. 15.10**).

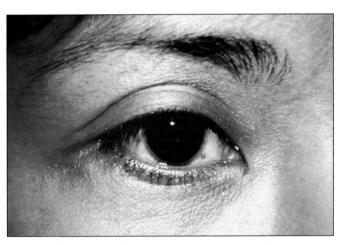

Figure 15.9 High, arched, semi-lunar crease on an Asian face.

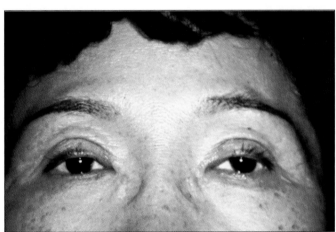

Figure 15.10 High sunken crease.

In a patient who has a pre-existent hollow below the superior orbital rim, further removal of preaponeurotic fat may exaggerate it into a prominent supratarsal sulcus with formation of multiple skin folds over the high crease (**Fig. 15.11**). In this situation, removal of more skin to eliminate these folds without addressing the problem of the high crease will usually lead to an even more obvious crease.

Problems associated with differences in crease depth between two lids are a more subtle aspect of asymmetry that may not be apparent to clinicians but can be an issue with some patients. The difference in softness (a soft crease readily disappears on downgaze, is considered 'dynamic', and imitates a physiologic crease) or harshness (a surgical-looking 'static' crease which does not shallow on downgaze and is readily apparent like a skin incision scar over the pretarsal skin) may be the combined result of interaction of the surgeon's variations in depth-placement of the crease-forming stitches between the two sides, versus the possible unequal responses of the patient's two eyelids in regards to crease formation (both in postoperative healing response as well as intrinsic levator function, which is an indication of the quality of levator muscle).

A crease may disappear relatively early (within 2 months) or late (after 6–9 months). In my experience, early disappearance, shallowing, or obliteration is most often due to insufficient clearing of the preaponeurotic platform of tissues along the superior tarsal border which results in an interference in the creation of a crease. It may occur due to other factors beyond the clinician's control – these include hemorrhage over the crease line, insect bite over the wound, acne and chalazion (stye) formation, cellulitis, and weak levator muscle. Undetected iatrogenic weakening of the levator aponeurosis can cause a segmental ptosis and poor crease formation.

Late disappearance of an otherwise well-formed crease can occur following significant weight gain and increase in the preseptal or sub-brow fat pads, or hypertrophy of the remaining central preaponeurotic (postseptal) or nasal fat pads. I recall one happy patient who in retrospect was probably borderline anorexic preoperatively, who had partial disappearance of one crease following resumption of her appetite after aesthetic improvement to her eyelids.

Problems associated with continuity are linked to the permanency issue discussed above, in the following fashion: if the crease is not well formed to its underlying aponeurosis in a continuous fashion, it may present as a discontinuous or broken crease and become evident soon after the surgery. A continuous crease may be well formed initially but then become obliterated, resulting in a shallow crease or no crease at all – in essence, a non-permanent crease. Or, it may break apart later, in a segmental fashion, giving a discontinuous but permanent crease. There appears to be a much higher incidence of disappearance of crease associated with the suture ligation methods (see Chapter 7).

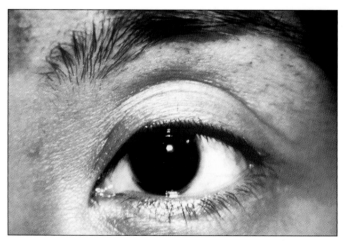

Figure 15.11 Prominent supratarsal sulcus with formation of multiple skin wrinkles over the high crease.

Patients who have multiple creases often may have undergone more than one surgery already. Pseudo-skin folds may become more apparent following creation of a dominant crease among multiple rudimentary creases or folds. The multiple creases may also arise from unpredictable scar formation in re-operative cases and in those patients who have undergone an excessive degree of dissection in the pretarsal region of the upper eyelid. In revision cases, it is vital to obtain close-up preoperative photographs of the crease in a frontal as well as downgaze position (to expose the crease), as well as documenting it in the patient's chart, drawing it and including it as part of the Informed Consent and disclosure/education to the patient. Any lack of understanding must be resolved prior to any procedure being offered.

The eyelids may look hollow from an excessive removal of fat pads. This may be further accentuated when the crease is placed higher than anatomically indicated. High anchoring of the crease line may also lead to a limited ability to elevate the lid upward (resulting in secondary ptosis) as well as cicatricial lagophthalmos (causing poor excursion of the upper lid margin) on downgaze.

At the opposite extreme, I have had the opportunity to work with several patients who desired to have their surgically placed crease reversed.

I will now go through some of the actual revision techniques for each of the suboptimal configurations.

By far the most often encountered revision problem is asymmetry. This includes creases that are unequal in height (**Fig. 15.12**), uneven in shape and continuity, shifting of the crease (downward migration of the crease; partial or complete obliteration of the crease) (Fig. 15.8), and fading of the medial one-third of the crease (**Fig. 15.13**).

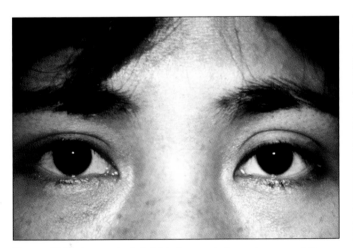

Figure 15.12 Asymmetry in height of crease between two upper lids.

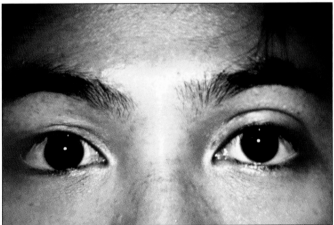

Figure 15.13 Fading of the medial one-third of the crease on each side, with asymmetry.

A. Excessively high crease

In evaluating patients in whom the eyelid crease on one side appears higher than on the other, often the higher crease is the abnormal one. It is essential to detect any acquired ptosis that may be present in this eyelid, as the levator aponeurosis often appears to have dehisced some of its lower terminal interdigitation and only has some of its more superior lid crease attachments left in this condition (**Fig. 15.14**). If such is the case, correction of the ptosis will eliminate the apparently higher crease without any attempts at repositioning of the crease.

A higher-than-normal crease can arise from inappropriate marking of the lines of incision, from inaccurate placement of the interrupted crease-forming sutures over the levator aponeurosis, or from persistent edema in the pretarsal plane. If a crease still appears high after an adequate time period (at least 6–9 months), the repair can be accomplished in the following fashion.

The lid with the higher crease is everted and the central height of the tarsus is measured. This measurement will serve as a reference, a point as to where the crease ought to be placed. When the tarsal height is transcribed on the skin side and is found to be closer to the eyelash line than the current crease, then the difference in millimeters of skin can be excised together with the previous incision scar, as long as there is not a shortage of skin that may prevent complete eyelid closure (**Fig. 15.15**). It is helpful to lyse any subcutaneous aponeurotic attachment along the superior edge of the incision. Any scar tissue that may overlie the aponeurotic attachment along the superior tarsal border should also be removed to allow for the reconstruction of the new crease.

If the transcribed tarsal height on the skin side is higher than your supposedly 'high' crease, then one should examine the contralateral upper lid crease to see if it has an excessively low crease.

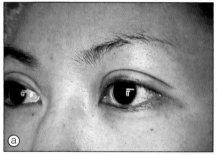

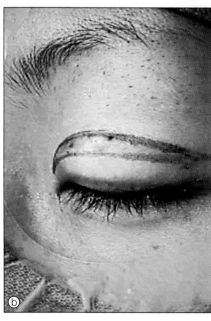

Figure 15.15 Excision of old incision line straddles the high crease in a revision case.

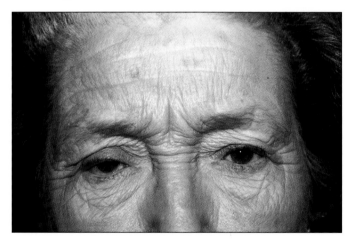

Figure 15.14 Relative acquired ptosis causing higher crease.

B. Excessively low crease

The challenge is greater in an excessively low crease (close to the lash margin). The correction is tailored as to whether there is any redundancy of skin.

For those who have some skin redundancy, I have found that the best method is still simple excision of the scar associated with this low crease, allowing it to heal, and then performing a subsequent crease procedure at least 6 months later. In my experience, simultaneous revision and construction of a new crease often results in suboptimal control of the crease height.

When the skin is taut and without any redundancy, simple excision is not possible since it may result in cicatricial ectropion or a prominent scar (**Fig. 15.16**). An acceptable option in a low crease with scarcity of skin is complete excision of the crease and the adjacent pretarsal skin, replacing it with a full-thickness skin graft and reforming the crease at the same time. This applies if the full-thickness skin graft covers the pretarsal region only. The patient should be forewarned that the crease will appear 'high' for at least 6 months.

Should the skin graft required span over the pretarsal region and the supratarsal region (**Fig. 15.17**), it is best to defer crease construction until several months after the skin grafting.

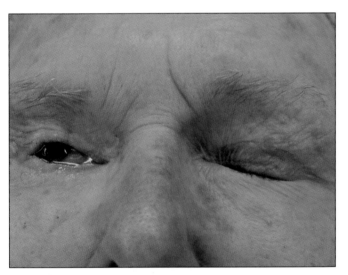

Figure 15.16 Caucasian with cicatricial lid retraction of right upper eyelid following upper blepharoplasty.

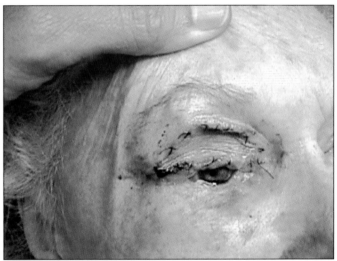

Figure 15.17 Same patient as in Figure 15.16, five days after full-thickness skin graft to the pretarsal zone.

C. Problems with permanency and/or continuity

Late obliteration of the crease includes patients with shallow crease, shifting of their crease, fading of the medial one-third of their crease, or obliteration of the entire crease (**Fig. 15.18**).

As long as there is some redundant healthy skin to work with, the Asian blepharoplasty technique described in Chapter 7 can be performed either partially or entirely along the width of the eyelid. I use spring Westcott scissors instead of the monopolar cautery needle tip to lyse the adhesion along the upper edge of the skin incision to reach the preaponeurotic space by first identifying the preaponeurotic fat pads. The most common findings at the time of surgery may include excessive subdermal scar and/or inadequate clearance of underlying orbicularis oculi, orbital septum, or fat pads (pretarsal or preaponeurotic) along the superior tarsal border at the junction of the pretarsal region and preaponeurotic space. The previous scar is excised and minimal skin is removed. The skin removed may be barely 1.0–1.5mm (**Fig. 15.19**).

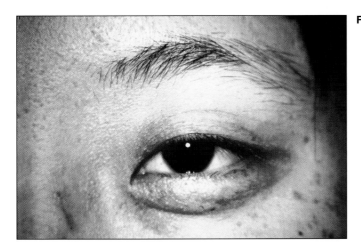

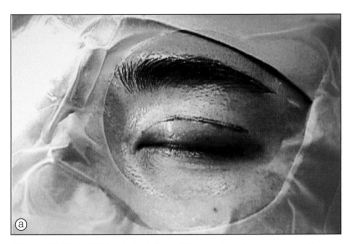

Figure 15.18 Late disappearance of left upper eyelid crease.

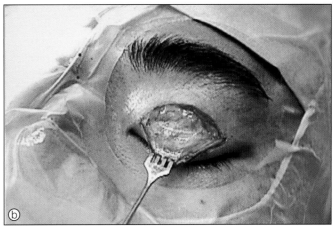

Figure 15.19 (a) Minimal straddling of the previous incision wound in a revision case with very tight skin.

Figure 15.19 (b) Westcott scissors were used to carefully lyse through the cicatrix of the orbicularis/septal complex along the superior edge of the incision wound.

A crease that is discontinuous will fare better if it is completely revised. Again, it is essential to trim away any underlying platform of scar tissue between the skin and healthy levator aponeurosis along the superior tarsal border.

Patients may present with an inadequate crease over the medial one-third (or less) of the upper lid (**Fig. 15.13**). This usually arises from insufficient subdermal attachment during the first operation and can be prevented by using at least three interrupted crease-forming sutures over the medial half of the crease (**Fig. 15.20**). It may also require more debulking of underlying soft tissue in that region in order to allow for a solid subcutaneous aponeurotic linkage.

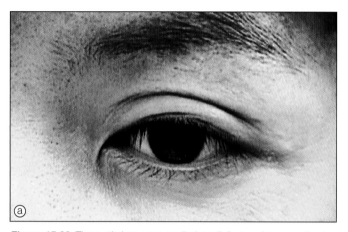 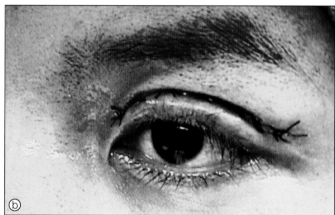

Figure 15.20 Three stitches were applied medially, to enhance an inadequately formed crease in a revision case involving a high crease.

D. Multiple creases

Patients may present with multiple creases over each eyelid. Such patients can be divided into two groups:

- those who had, for example, multiple faint creases to start with, but who end up with several competing and prominent creases; and

- those who were without any crease to start with.

Patients in the former group may have had several rudimentary creases (**Fig. 15.21**) or one noticeable crease with several less obvious ones at the outset but nevertheless finish up with several even more prominent creases. In my experience, this phenomenon is seen in those patients who have undergone vigorous dissection in the pretarsal and preaponeurotic space, or who have undergone excessive removal of pretarsal tissues in an attempt to 'remove all pretarsal fat', or overzealous removal of preaponeurotic fat pad. These multiple creases tend to be low, occurring in the pretarsal region.

In such cases, the anatomical based method of Asian blepharoplasty using the tarsal height as a guide to crease placement is still the best way to 'condense' several creases into a relatively more dominant crease, provided that there is redundant skin to work with. Frequently, several closely spaced creases can be completely excised with good results. When there is severe skin shortage in a patient who presents with multiple creases, functional correction of the skin shortage using a full-thickness skin graft takes precedence over the aesthetic aspect. The redundant creases may be excised when performing the skin graft, and a secondary procedure carried out later to form the crease.

With regard to the subtype of patients who were without any crease to start with but end up with multiple creases, in my experience almost all result from excessive removal of preaponeurotic fat pads. They frequently have had excessively high placement of their main crease, and the redundant creases are all high in the supratarsal region. In my observation, these 'creases' are really the interspaces between multiple folds of skin left behind from excessive removal of preaponeurotic fat pads (see Fig. 15.5).

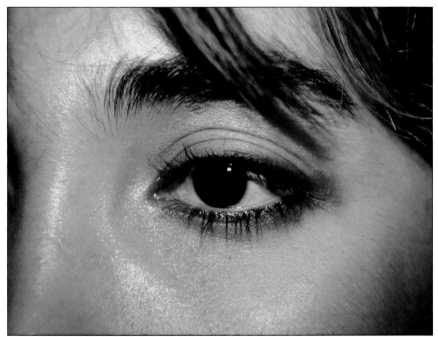

Figure 15.21 A patient who has never had surgery, illustrating the presence of multiple rudimentary creases.

E. Hollow supratarsal sulcus, with or without multiple creases

Hollowness of the sulcus may be pre-existent but exaggerated with removal of preaponeurotic fat, or arise iatrogenically from surgery.

In the medical literature, there is a myriad of corrections – placement of methylmethacrylate implants in the supratarsal sulcus, injections of collagen and silicone, and autogenous free fat grafts have all been tried. I have not found any good, permanent solution to correcting the problem of excessive removal of preaponeurotic fat. The use of a dermis–fat graft, interspacing it in the superior conjunctival fornix, has been used with some success.

For patients who have a hollow sulcus and multiple folds with adequate redundancy of skin, I offer them the option of converting the multiple folds into a single tarsal height-based crease.

F. Half-moon crease

Patients with a semi-lunar crease configuration are often unhappy. The primary surgeon may have designed the crease based on a traditional blepharoplasty technique, placing the crease such that the widest separation to the lash margin occurs in the mid-portion of the eyelid, with the ends of the crease tapering down towards each canthus. The result is often a 'round-eye' look. It is especially evident on Asians since they tend to have a smaller eyelid fissure width. The same 10mm separation from crease to lash line, arching towards each canthus, will subtend a greater arc angle in Asians than in Caucasians, as Asians have smaller eyelid fissure width (**Fig. 15.22**) – hence, a greater degree of 'round eye'. This is the exact opposite of what most Asians desire. By contrast, a nasally tapered crease, or a parallel crease, will make the eyelid fissure appear wider in its horizon dimension, more 'open-ended', and larger in its apparent vertical dimension (**Fig. 15.23**).

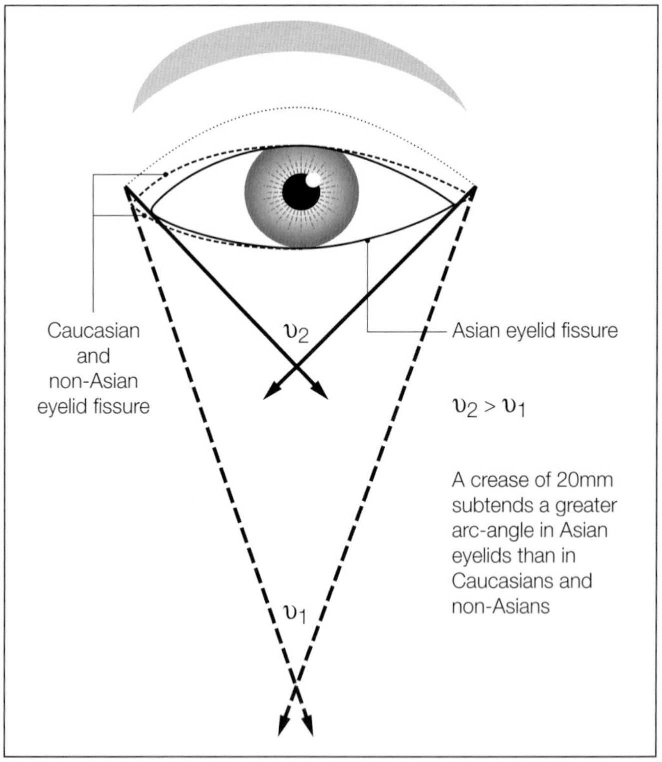

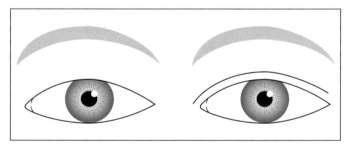

Figure 15.23 The visual effect of a crease over the left upper eyelid, with the eyelid fissure drawn exactly of the same dimension. In reality, single eyelids (without crease) often have a small fold of skin overhanging and therefore the fissure size is even smaller as measured vertically before any procedure. When the excess is artfully removed and a crease applied, it adds a great degree to the aesthetic appeal. (Reproduced with permission from Chen WP. Asian blepharoplasty: a surgical atlas. Newton: Butterworth–Heinemann; 1995: 3.)

Caucasian and non-Asian eyelid fissure

v_2

Asian eyelid fissure

$v_2 > v_1$

A crease of 20mm subtends a greater arc-angle in Asian eyelids than in Caucasians and non-Asians

v_1

Figure 15.22 The smaller Asian eyelid fissure subtends a larger angle with a given width of crease versus that which occurs in a Caucasian eyelid. (Reproduced with permission from Chen WP. Asian blepharoplasty: a surgical atlas. Newton: Butterworth–Heinemann; 1995: 96.)

Surgical solution:

A tarsal height-based technique of Asian blepharoplasty is preferred, using a crease height of 6.5–8.0mm, with a nasally tapered or parallel crease configuration. The open-sky skin incision approach allows for accurate placement of sutures over the aponeurosis, and provides a greater control over crease formation.

1. Semi-lunar crease ≤10mm from lid margin

When confronted with a semi-lunar crease, as long as the maximum height of the abnormal crease to be revised is 10mm or less, the central 50% of the crease may be moved down in the following fashion.

(a) For the patient with some redundancy of skin

After 6 to 9 months from the last surgery, the central tarsal height is measured and transcribed onto the eyelid skin. The segment of skin between this preferred crease line and the undesirable, higher semicircular crease is marked out (usually not more than 2–3mm). The central 50% of the semi-lunar crease is excised by removing the 2mm strip of skin between it

and the preferred lower crease (**Fig. 15.24**). This has the net effect of converting the crease into a nasally tapered configuration. A mild degree of undermining is performed along the upper edge of the semi-lunar crease, to free any subcutaneous attachment of septum and levator aponeurosis. The medial 25% of the semi-lunar crease now becomes the nasally tapered portion of the preferred crease; the central 50% is re-formed at a lower level in a parallel continuous crease, while the lateral one-quarter of the semi-lunar crease is excised and revised so that it is either parallel or slightly flared upward by deliberately anchoring it higher than it was. This is facilitated by undermining the subcutaneous tissue around the lateral canthal region.

The challenge arises when there is very little skin between the lateral portion of the semi-lunar crease and the lateral canthus. I find it more effective to excise the lateral one-quarter of the crease and perform simple plastic closure; then return 6 months later to perform a lateral crease revision.

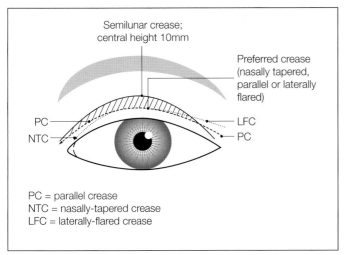

Figure 15.24 Surgical conversion of a semi-lunar crease (solid line) to a narrower parallel crease (hyphenated line) or a nasally tapered crease (dotted line). (Reproduced with permission from Chen WP. Asian blepharoplasty: a surgical atlas. Newton: Butterworth–Heinemann; 1995: 97.)

(b) For those patients with skin shortage

The semi-lunar crease is not easily revised unless the crease with its underlying scar and the skin between the semi-lunar crease and the new crease (based on tarsal height) are completely excised. Full-thickness skin grafts are used to correct the skin shortage above the proposed crease and to allow for reconstruction of a lower crease (**Figs 15.25a & b**). The crease is to be formed at the junction of the pretarsal skin and the skin graft.

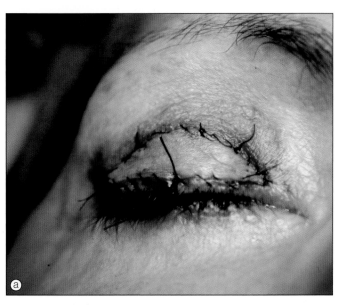

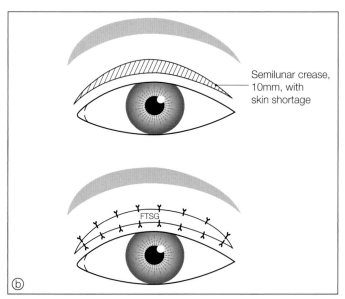

Figure 15.25 (a) Shortage of skin in a patient with a semi-lunar high crease. The segment has been excised and the crease shape converted to a lower parallel configuration. (Reproduced with permission from Chen WP. Asian blepharoplasty: a surgical atlas. Newton: Butterworth–Heinemann; 1995: 99.)

Figure 15.25 (b) A full-thickness skin graft is then added over the recipient area of the lid. The new crease is to be formed at the junction of the pretarsal skin and the lower border of the skin graft. (Reproduced with permission from Chen WP. Asian blepharoplasty: a surgical atlas. Newton: Butterworth–Heinemann; 1995: 99.)

2. Semi-lunar crease >10mm from lid margin

A much more challenging situation exists when the semi-lunar crease is more than 10mm from the lid margin. I have seen patients with creases as high as 12–15mm (**Fig. 15.26**).[7] The correction of this crease involves working closer to the eyebrow's thicker dermis, with less camouflage and a greater chance for hypertrophic scarring.

On the rare occasion when there is some redundant skin in conjunction with a highly placed semilunar crease (>10mm), one may try the same steps as described in subsection 1(a).

Unfortunately, most of these patients have undergone excessive skin removal and present with little skin left for plastic reconstruction. The repair will require a full-thickness skin graft as detailed in subsection 1(b), noting that the upper edge of the skin graft will be quite conspicuous.

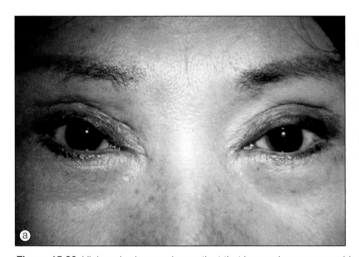 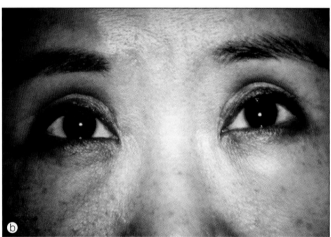

Figure 15.26 High-arched crease in a patient that has undergone upper blepharoplasty.

G. Removal of surgically placed crease

My most challenging clinical cases have been the few patients who want their surgically placed crease completely reversed. In these patients, I have tried to remove an existing surgically created crease using a variety of methods, some with better results than others:

■ Excision of crease and scar, application of traction sutures inferiorly (reverse Frost sutures) – minimum improvement.

■ Subcutaneous lysis of adhesions using small tenotomy scissors – minimum improvement.

■ Excision of crease and scar, with interposition of orbicularis fibers to block the aponeurotic–subdermal attachment – mild improvement.

■ Excision of crease and scar, and closure of the wound with $\frac{1}{4}$" Steri-Strip tape; patients are encouraged to avoid looking up during the first week (avoid contraction of the levator aponeurosis) – mild improvement.

■ Excision of crease and scar, recession of the levator aponeurotic muscle, and placement of autologous temporalis fascia (**Fig. 15.27**) – significant improvement.

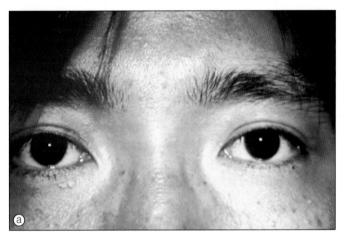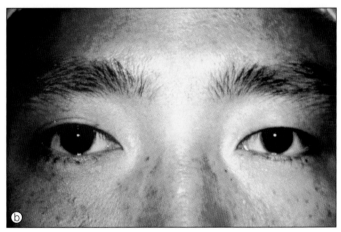

Figure 15.27 Pre- and postoperative view of a man who elected to have crease reversal. Temporalis fascia was used to obliterate the crease. The result was satisfactory, although a faint but noticeable crease is still seen over the lateral portion of the right upper lid.

We will now discuss some of the surgical solutions I have used on complicated revision cases: **Figures** **15.28–15.57** illustrate 30 patients with revision and challenging crease management problems.

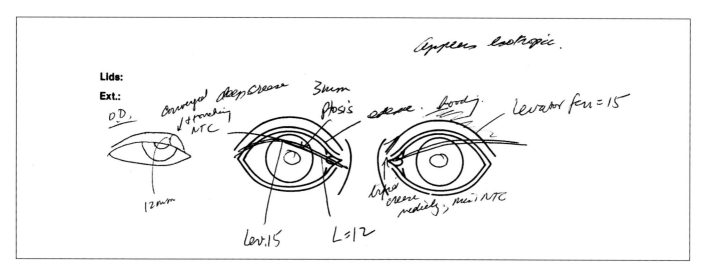

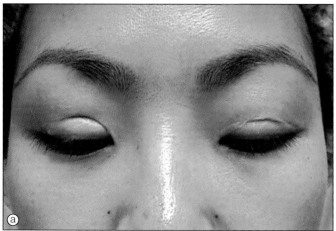
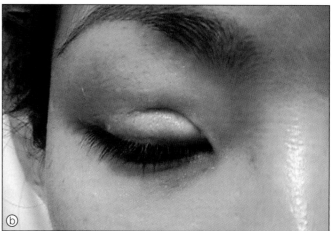

Figure 15.28

Commentary:

Had surgery 4 years ago and a second time a year prior to being seen.

Right upper lid – deep crease, converging and touching NTC, with 3mm ptosis.

Left upper lid – medial bifurcation of crease as it approaches the medial canthal fold.

Levator function: R 12mm, L 15mm.

Appears esotropic.

Body height: 5' 0".

Intraoperatively: Right side harsh and static 12mm crease, bound down.

Tarsus measured 6mm.

Designed 6mm NTC.

Incision with No. 15 blade, then used blunted-tipped Westcott spring scissors to lyse adhesions along superior edge until preaponeurotic fat is seen (no true septum left).

Used cutting cautery to remove scar and redundancy along preaponeurotic platform, plus removal of 8-0 nylon buried sutures that were used for crease formation.

Formed crease with 6-0 and 7-0 silk sutures that were removed after 5 days.

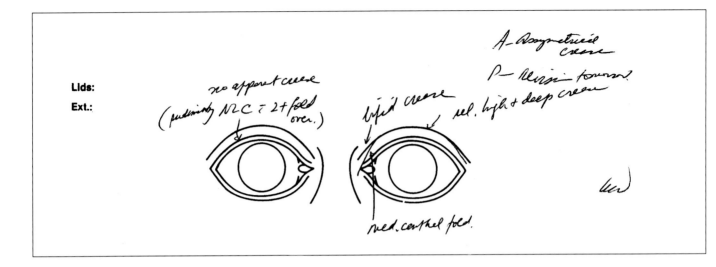

Lids:

Ext.:

no apparent crease
(preliminary NLC = 2+ fold over.)

bifid crease

med. canthal fold.

A- Asymmetrical crease

P- Revision tomorrow

rel. high + deep crease

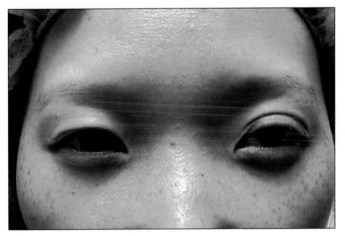

Figure 15.29

Commentary:
Patient from out of State.
7 years status post lid crease. RUL hooded and rudimentary crease. LUL has high crease with bifid ending both corners.
Intraoperatively: Tarsus measured 7mm.
Designed NTC O.U.
RUL – removed 2mm skin and orbicularis. Used scissors to go through upper edge of incision, staying beveled to reach preaponeurotic plane.
LUL – eliminated bifid crease, removed buried nylon sutures.

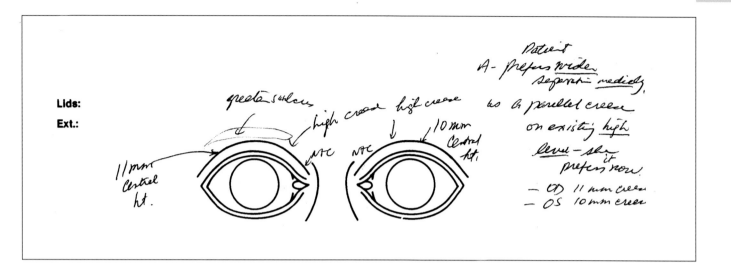

Lids:
Ext.:

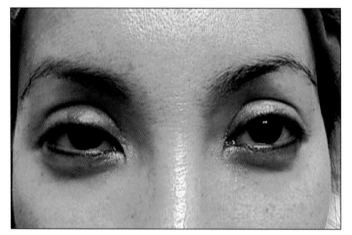

Figure 15.30

Commentary:
47-year-old patient with first surgery 20 years ago coupled with 'W-plasty'; then revision 12 years ago. Intraoperatively: Prominent medial aponeurotic fat as well as nasal fat pad. Removed fat pads. Use 6-0 Vicryl to fixate inferior orbicularis to levator and then superior orbicularis; keep suture knot buried.

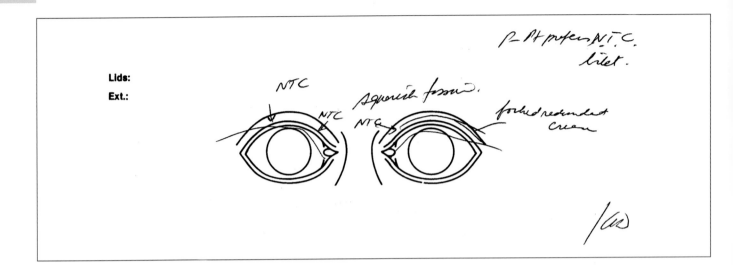

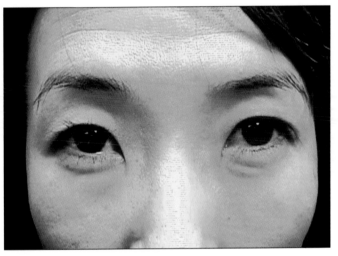

Figure 15.31

Commentary:

33 year old who has never had surgery but has used adhesive tapes since 17 years of age to create crease. Shows mild sulcus. Practices yoga and kick-boxing. Intraoperatively: Tarsus measured 8.5mm. I used 8mm as lower line of incision Designed NTC, included 2mm skin.

Preserved all preaponeurotic fat and reposited it within the sulcus. Excised strip of myocutaneous flap. Formed crease with 6-0 and 7-0 silk sutures, which were removed at 1 week.

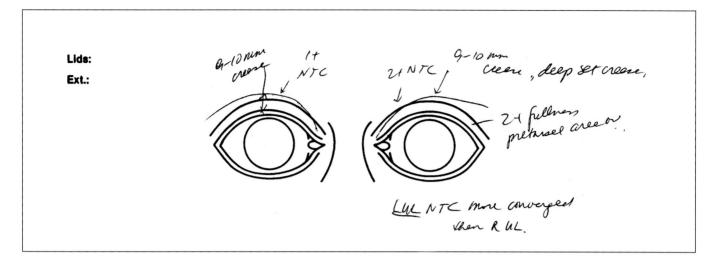

Lids:
Ext.:

9–10 mm crease   1+ NTC   2+ NTC   9–10 mm crease, deep set crease,   2+ fullness pretarsel area on.

LUL NTC more converged than R UL.

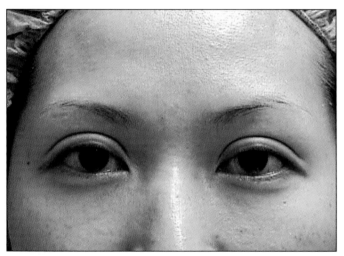

Figure 15.32

Commentary:

29-year-old housewife. Had surgery at 18 years of age in Korea.

RUL 9–10mm crease position OU and appears deepset. Has moderate fullness over pretarsal area LUL is more converged medially than that of the RUL.

Intraoperatively: Her tarsus was only 5.5–6.0mm. RUL crease measured 11mm, LUL at 10mm. Designed 8.5mm parallel crease over RUL with some tapering medially; and 8mm over LUL in attempt to equalize two asymmetric high creases.

Use blunt scissors to reach preaponeurotic space superiorly. Large amount of cicatrix over preseptal as well as pretarsal zones. Excised strip of myocutaneous flap OU. Excised strip of pretarsal inferior orbicularis muscle to reduce fullness. Checked levator's excursion on the table and appeared full OU.

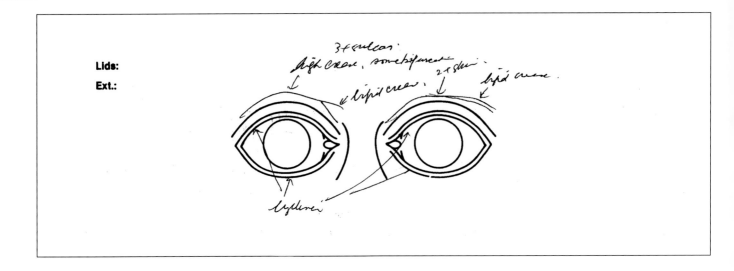

Lids:

Ext.:

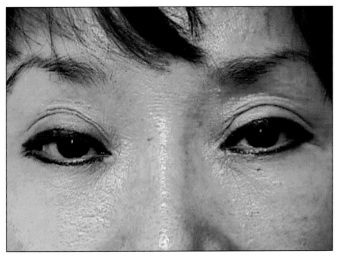

Figure 15.33

Commentary:

55 year old had four-lid blepharoplasty 10 years prior in Hawaii. Has high bifid semi-lunar creases OU, measured to be 10–11mm in sulcus.

Intraoperatively: Designed parallel crease OU at 7.5mm (tarsus measured 7mm).

Excised old crease with 1mm clear skin superior to it, with the lower skin incision edge at 7.5mm.

Found very attenuated levator muscle with fatty infiltration.

Formed parallel crease.

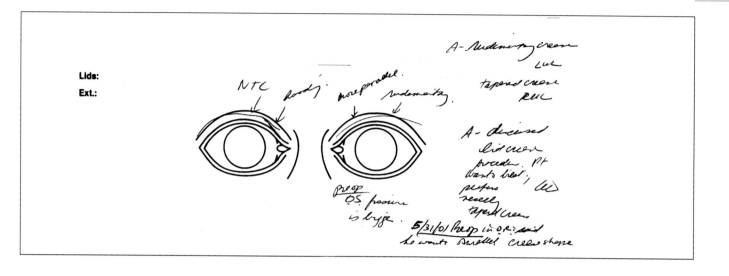

Lids:

Ext.:

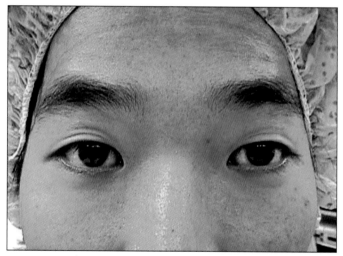

Figure 15.34

Commentary:
29 year old had crease procedure 9 years prior – stitch method alone with adjustment twice. LUL has no crease. RUL has shallow NTC. Patient prefers parallel crease.
Intraoperatively: Very vascular. Removed nylon sutures from along the superior tarsal border. Used 6-0 silk and 6-0 Prolene with significant attachment towards the levator aponeurosis.

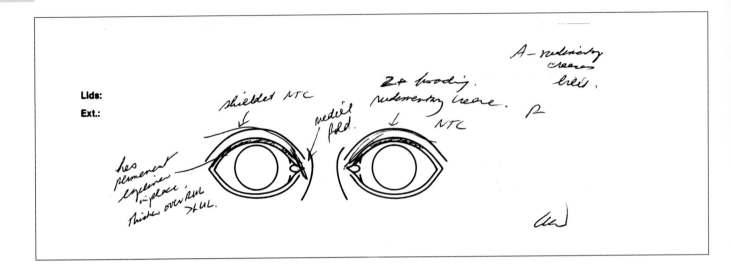

Lids:

Ext.:

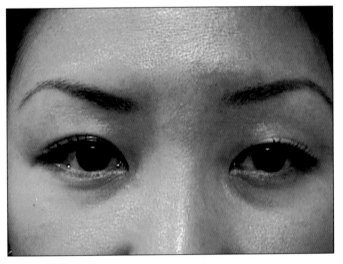

Figure 15.35

Commentary:

25 year old. RUL with rudimentary crease. LUL none. Right side has medial canthal fold. Has permanent eyeliner in place and is thicker over the right compared with the left.

Intraoperatively: Tarsus measured 7mm; thick skin, acniform.

Preaponeurotic fat appears mosaic and ill-defined, creeping to a point well below the superior tarsal border, interlaced with fibrotic strands.

Used 6-0 silk and 6-0 Prolene.

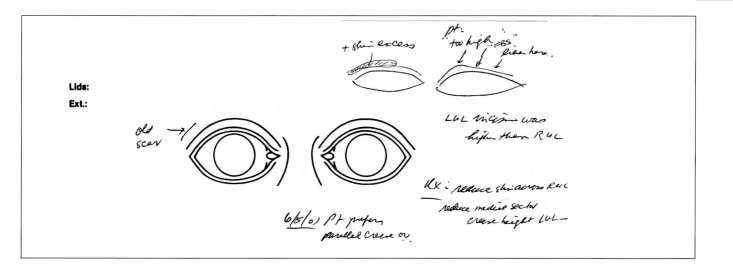

Lids:

Ext.:

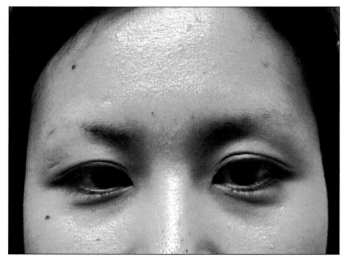

Commentary:

36 year old.

Three years status post lid crease procedure. Currently has shielded crease over RUL, and LUL has wider separation from lid margin than the RUL. Wants parallel crease.

Intraoperatively: Designed 7mm crease height to encompass RUL scar. Excised moderate amount of preaponeurotic fat from RUL as well as inferior orbicularis strip.

LUL – Reduced the crease height medially. Fat not as excessive and therefore only reduced some with bipolar wetfield cautery. Excised inferior orbicularis strip. Closed with 6-0 silk. Inspection revealed crease still high. Take down and re-excised 1mm skin from lower edge. Result was more symmetrical look.

Figure 15.36

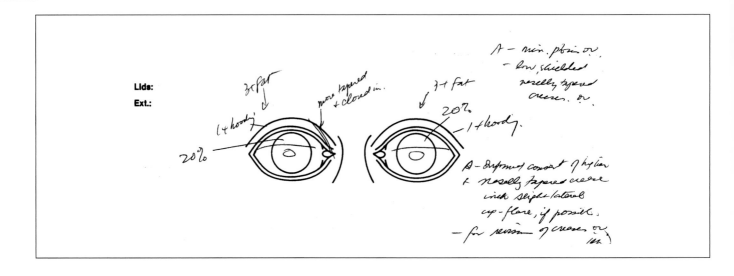

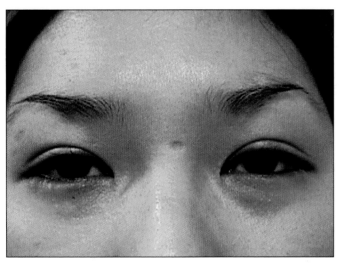

Figure 15.37

Commentary:

22-year-old Asian. 5' 7" with low-set NTC, partially shielded. 2mm cornea covered OU. Using cotton-tip application, patient indicated a crease height closer to 9–10mm as being her preferred configuration. Desires slight lateral up-flare.

Intraoperatively: Used 8mm to define an NTC; including 1mm of scar adhesion. Upon reaching preaponeurotic space, fat was not abundant. Excised strip of skin/muscle/scar tissues, as well as preseptal strip of orbicularis above and along the superior tarsal border. Designed slight lateral up-flare.

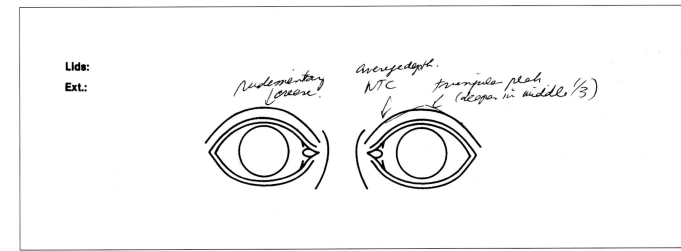

Lids:
Ext.:

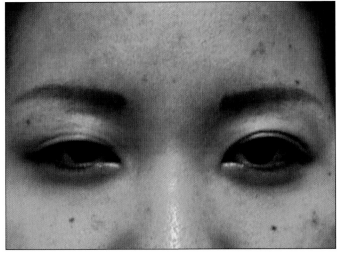

Figure 15.38

Commentary:

24 year old had lid crease procedure in Hong Kong 8 years prior. RUL crease never did form and is now shallow; LUL crease is deeper but central portion slightly peaked.

Desired NTC.

Intraoperatively: RUL tarsus measured 6.5mm. Used 7mm to design an NTC. Resected scar tissues, no fat. Used 6-0 and 7-0 silk.

LUL – 'square-well' excision of strip of scar tissue along superior tarsal border. Mid-section underwent some dissection superiorly to make it less fibrosed down to the aponeurosis. Re-formed smooth NTC with good result.

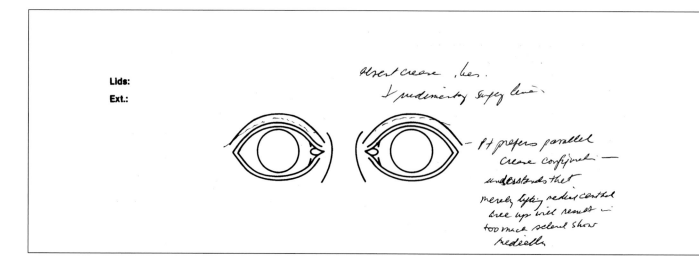

Lids:

Ext.:

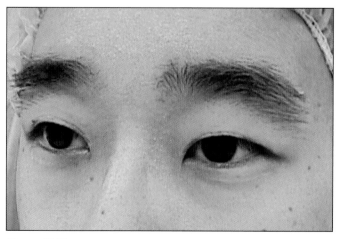

Figure 15.39

Commentary:

Male patient. Nine years previously had lid crease procedure. The crease did not fold in well by the end of the first week. Revised 2 months later with same finding. Has very faint rudimentary line OU. Patient wanted the medial one-third of the crease to be lifted higher. However, this would lead to a triangular or rectangular look. After careful discussion, the patient chose a parallel crease.

Intraoperatively: Tarsus measured 8mm. We designed a 7mm parallel crease. Lysed scar tissues along the upper incisional edge, through orbicularis. Observed amorphous fat plastered against levator muscle.

After the skin muscle flap was trimmed, there were still remnants of preseptal tissues along the superior tarsal border; as the patient looks up, this redundant tissue would bunch up and make the crease look low and 'rope-like'. This was then excised to show a clean insertion of the aponeurosis along the superior tarsal border. The lower skin edge was pulled up and united with aponeurosis along the superior tarsal border, forming a nice parallel 7mm crease.

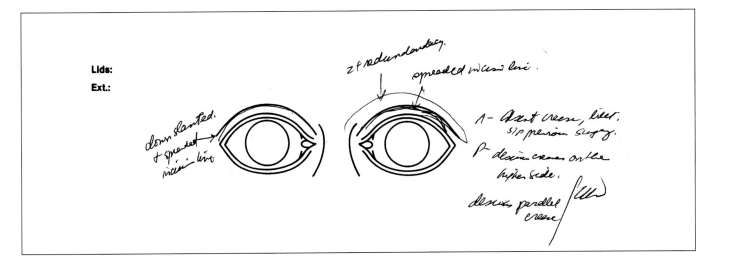

Lids:
Ext.:

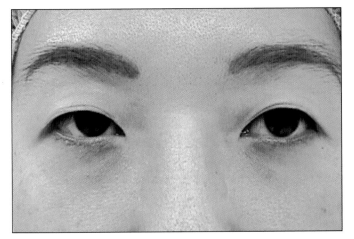

Figure 15.40

Commentary:

30 year old who was 10 years after external incision crease procedure. The lateral extent of the RUL appears downslant towards the lateral canthus. The incisional line has spread over the left side. Desires parallel crease to be of above-average height. Intraoperatively: Tarsus measured 8mm. Used a parallel 8mm incision line, included 2.5mm skin. Very vascular orbicularis oculi muscle. Preaponeurotic fat pad protrudes inferiorly over the lateral half and required partial excision. The rest of the fat seemed spread out and plastered down. Formed crease with 6-0 and 7-0 silk.

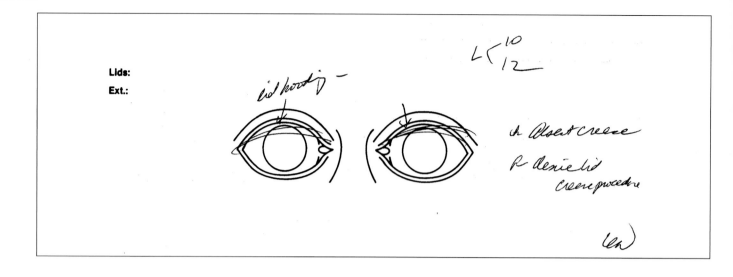

Lids:

Ext.:

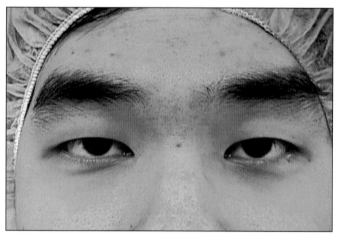

Figure 15.41

Commentary:

24-year-old male was told that crease procedure will not be successful due to weak muscle.

Patient is 6-feet tall and has mild hooding.

Levator function: RUL 10mm, LUL 12 mm.

Wanted 'natural Asian crease'.

Intraoperatively: Tarsus measured 8mm. However, the lid margin distance to his lower border of the eyebrow is narrow and therefore opted to design a 6.5mm minimally tapered, almost parallel crease. Orbicularis was soft, fluctuant, and vascular.

Opened the orbital septum and patient had large amount of otherwise unsuspected preaponeurotic fat pad. Removed 80% of this in this particular case. Excised myocutaneous flap. Formed crease with 6-0 and 7-0 silk.

Lids:

Ext.:

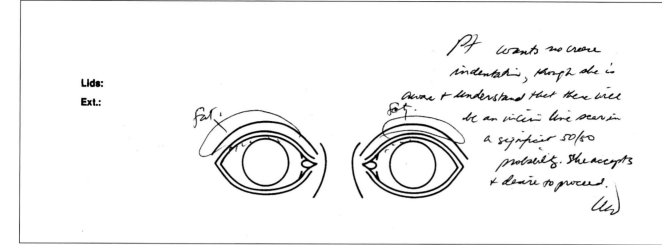

Pt wants no crease indentation, though she is aware + understand that there will be an incision line scar in a significant 50/50 probability. She accepts + desire to proceed.

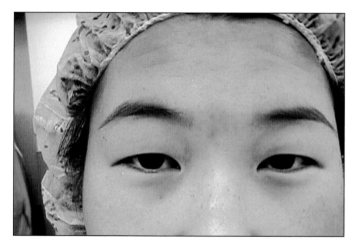

Figure 15.42

Commentary:
19 year old. Heavy upper lid hooding with fat. Some brow action. Wants to have hooding and fat removed but does not want crease formation. Height is 5' 3".

Intraoperatively: Tarsus measured 7mm. Used hyaluronidase in local injection. Made lower incision line at 5mm and included 3mm of skin in a parallel configuration. After using blade through skin, used cutting cautery with very fine tip to traverse through the upper edge of the orbicularis. Reached septum and opened it. Excised 80% of prolapsing preaponeurotic fat. Excised myocutaneous strip that consisted mostly of skin, leaving behind half of the orbicularis along the superior tarsal border. Closed orbicularis to orbicularis with 6-0 Vicryl. Skin closed with 6-0 nylon in a running fashion, taking bites of skin only. No interrupted sutures were used on the skin.

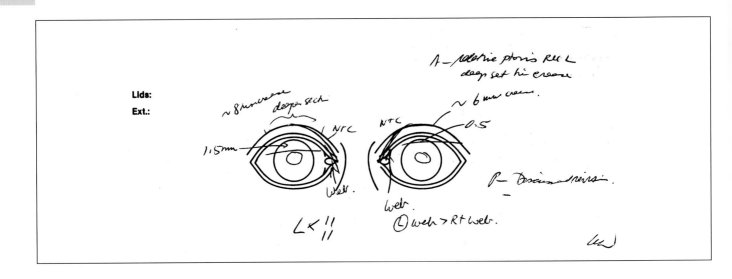

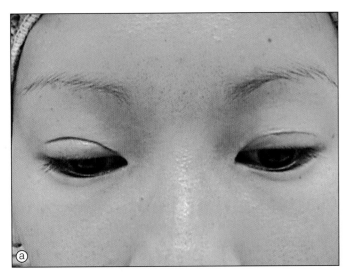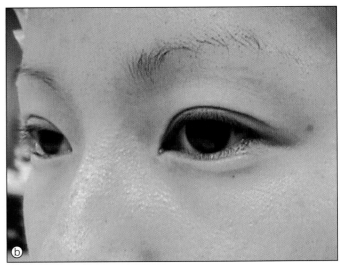

Figure 15.43

Commentary:

22 year old.

Four years status post lid crease procedure and attempted ptosis repair of the right upper lid. RUL crease is deep set and crease height was 8mm, with 1.5mm of cornea covered. LUL has deep-set 6mm crease, 0.5mm cornea is covered.

Intraoperatively: Measured right tarsus and it was only 5.5mm, probably had tarsectomy. LUL tarsus measured 7mm.

RUL: Very vascular. Created 7mm NTC and included 2mm skin. Found three blue nylon stitches, scarred levator/tarsus junction. Performed external resection of aponeurosis, measuring 3mm (see Chapter 12). Dissected epitarsally to smooth out already swollen tarsal area. Formed crease with 6-0 and 7-0 silk.

LUL: Set crease height at 7mm also, and NTC. Found three nylon stitches and removed them. Excised 1.5mm skin–muscle strip. Formed crease.

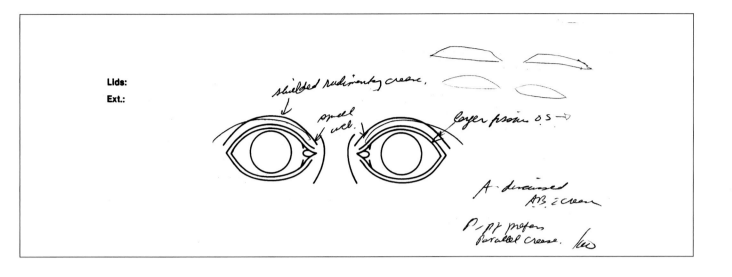

Lids:

Ext.:

shielded rudimentary crease.

small ucl.

layer psom O.S →

A. discussed AB = crease

P. pt prefers parallel crease.

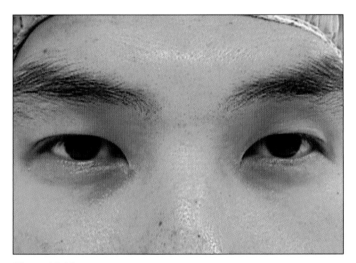

Figure 15.44

Commentary:

36 year old with shielded rudimentary crease over both sides. Small but noticeable medial canthal web. Has rectangular (trapezoidal) appearance to palpebral fissures. Patient was informed of likely eye shape change if has procedure. Patient wanted parallel crease. He is 6 feet tall.

Intraoperatively: Tarsus measured 8mm. However, short distance from upper lid margin to inferior edge of brow. Therefore, despite the fact that he is tall, I used 7.5mm and designed a parallel crease.

RUL – large amount of preaponeurotic fat excised OU. The inferior orbicularis area is infiltrated with fat and is trimmed. Medial canthal web acceptable and untouched.

LUL– same as RUL. Medial canthal fold here had small dog-ear that required excision. Used 7-0 silk to close this area.

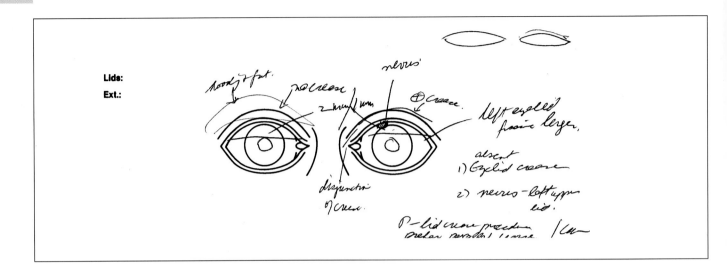

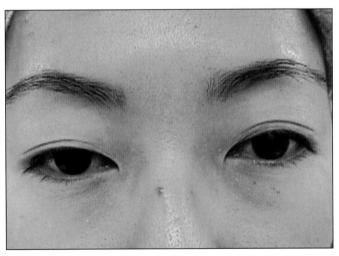

Figure 15.45

Commentary:

32 year old who used eyelid tape bilaterally to help crease formation. RUL crease rudimentary, with 2mm cornea covered. LUL has crease with competing folds and dysjunction medially. LUL margin covers 1mm of cornea. Height 5' 5". Prefers parallel crease.

Intraoperatively: Tarsus measured 7mm. Used 7mm to design parallel crease. Debulked preaponeurotic fat. Used McCord's crease fixation method with 6-0 Vicryl in addition to usual 6-0 and 7-0 silk method.

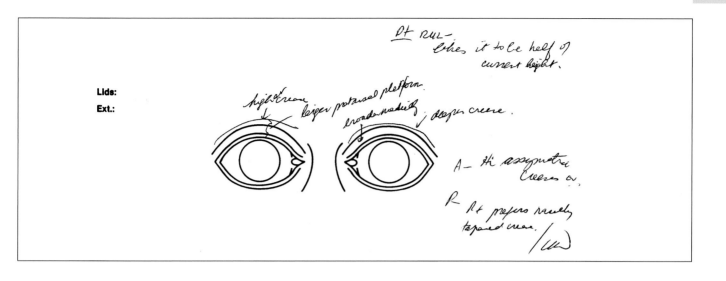

Lids:

Ext.:

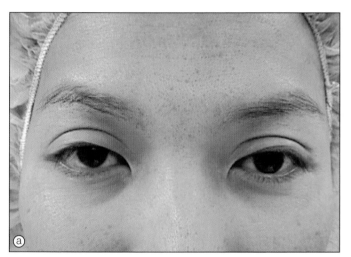

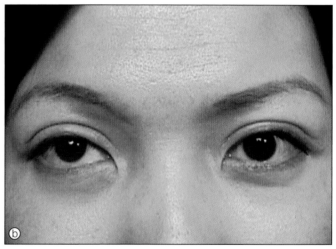

Figure 15.46

Commentary:

36 year old who was 10 years after first crease procedure. RUL had 12mm crease height with broad medial portion; LUL had 14mm deep crease. Height is 5' 7".

Intraoperatively: Her tarsus measured 7mm. Used 8mm as crease.

Included 3mm skin segment. Opened preaponeurotic plane with Westcott scissors along the upper edge. No fat seen. Formed crease with 6-0 and 7-0 silk.

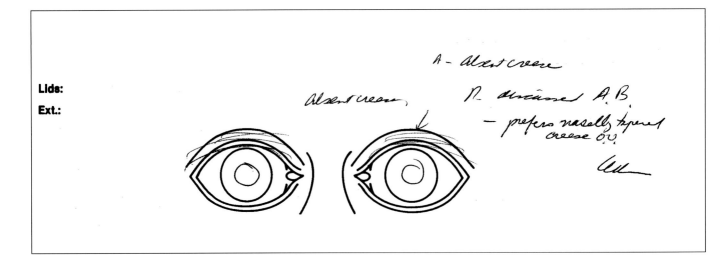

Lids:

Ext.:

A - Absent crease

Absent crease,

R. discuss A, B.

— prefers nasally tapered crease OU.

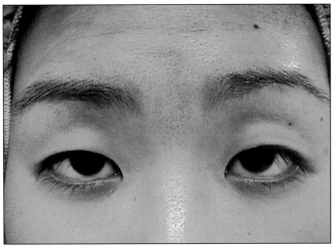

Figure 15.47

Commentary:
18 year old with absent crease. Prefers nasally tapered crease. Height is 5' 2".
Intraoperatively: Tarsus measured 8mm. Used 7mm to design crease, included 2mm skin – very spongy pretarsal tissues. Has layer of fatty tissue along superior tarsal border which was excised but without well-defined pre-aponeurotic fat.
RUL crease appeared high centrally at end of case and this area was adjusted down by excising 1mm of skin along the lower edge over the central two-thirds of the lid width.

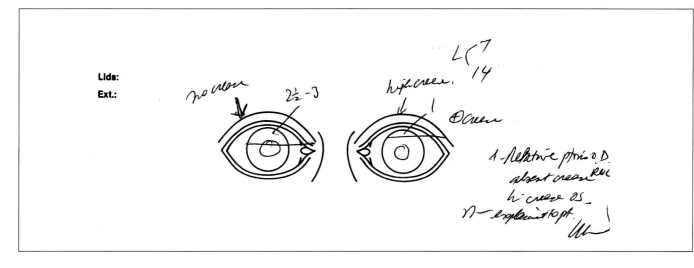

Lids:
Ext.:

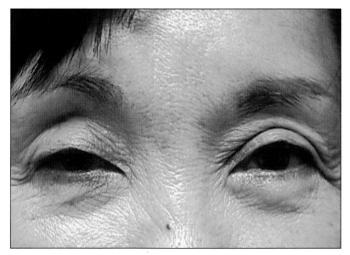

Figure 15.48

Commentary:

66 year old. Right upper lid with 3mm ptosis, hollow sulcus, and absent crease.

LUL has high crease. Levator function: RUL 7mm, LUL 14 mm.

Intraoperatively: RUL has had previous tarsectomy-type procedure. Applied frontal nerve block. Performed lysis of adhesion along the superior edge of the skin incision. Levator was extrememly attenuated. The aponeurosis was elevated from underlying conjuntiva and then 10mm resected. The edge of the muscle was then advanced and re-anastomosed inferiorly along the STB using 6-0 Vicryl. Formed crease with multiple 6-0 and 7-0 silk. LUL – created six crease line incisions, then dissected upwards towards cicatrix to reach preaponeurotic plane. Resected the old cicatrix and fragment of skin between it and the new lower edge of the crease incision.

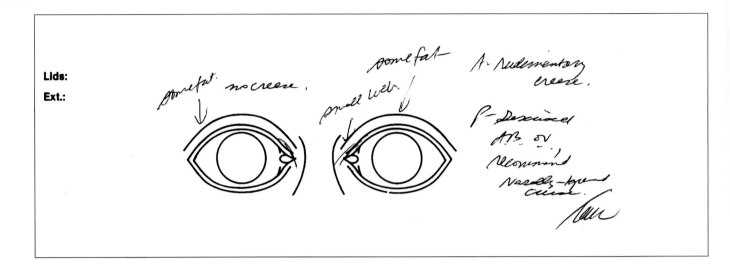

Lids:

Ext.:

some fat. no crease.

some fat

small web.

A. rudimentary crease.

P. Desired AB ov. Recommend Nasally-tapered crease.

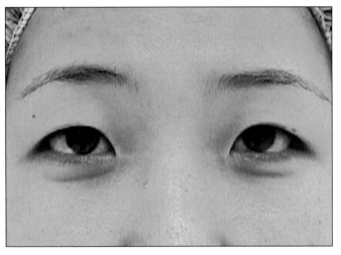

Figure 15.49

Commentary:

23 year old with rudimentary crease OU. The upper lid margin appeared to peak over the medial one-third. Desired nasally tapered crease.

I performed Asian blepharoplasty. Five years later, patient now in residency training; creases have disappeared from both eyes. Eyelids now appear just as full, even though first procedure had involved preaponeurotic fat excision.

Intraoperatively: Tarsus measured 6.5mm. Used 7mm to mark crease. Had very soft fluctuant pretarsal and preseptal tissues. Had amorphous downwardly migrated preseptal (sub-brow) fat, which was disrupting the crease formation. This was reposited superiorly. Excised scar and myocutaneous flap. Formed crease with 6-0 and 7-0 silk in a nasally tapered configuration.

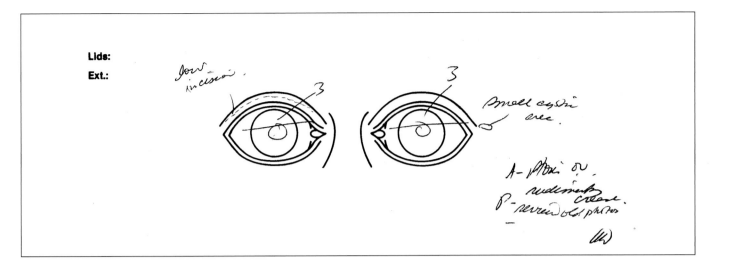

Lids:
Ext.:

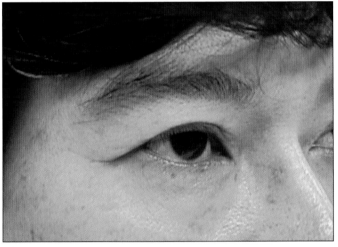

Figure 15.50

Commentary:

46 year old from South America. Two years ago had undergone upper blepheroplasty with incision placed 3mm from lash margin. Now has recurrent hooding such that the crease is shielded and there is dark-colored skin along incision. Wanted parallel crease. Lid margin rests 3mm down on cornea. Intraoperatively: Upper lid skin appears short prior to intervention. Used 5mm parallel line to incise skin, then lysed along the superior skin edge until large amount of preseptal and preaponeurotic fat was seen. Made a small trough above the superior tarsal border, just enough to facilitate skin closure. No skin excision at all.

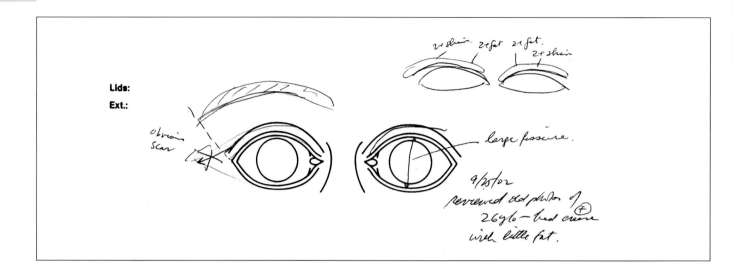

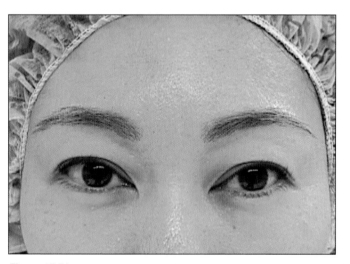

Figure 15.51

Commentary:

40 year old from South-East Asia, wanting to have upper eyelid and fat removal.

Had prominent eye fissures, mild fat, and some hooding. Wanted 'natural, conservative nasally tapered crease'.

Intraoperatively: Tarsus 7.5mm. Designed crease with 2mm skin. Excised portion of preaponeurotic fat bilaterally.

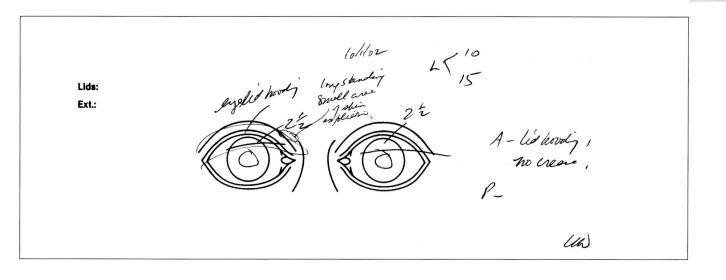

Lids:

Ext.:

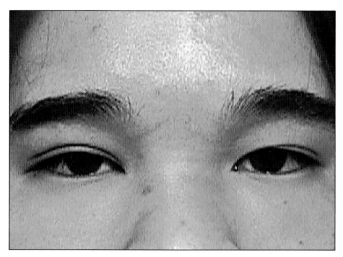

Figure 15.52

Commentary:

18 year old complains of intermittent or absence of crease over the right side. Height is 5' 7". Intraoperatively: Tarsus measured to be 7.5mm. His rudimentary crease appears to be at 7mm; therefore designed 7mm NTC, plus 2mm of skin. Fat was reduced with bipolar cautery. Excised orbicularis along the path of the superior tarsal border. Medially there was some web formation and these were reduced and the crease anchored deeper here with 6-0 silk to prevent web formation medially.

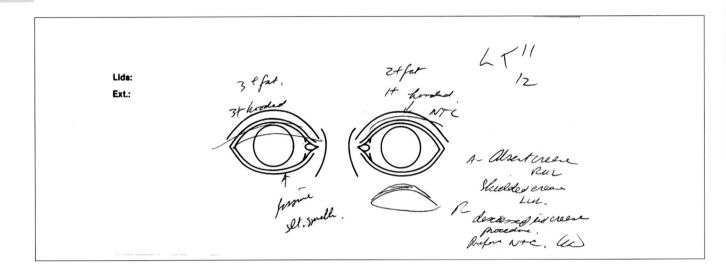

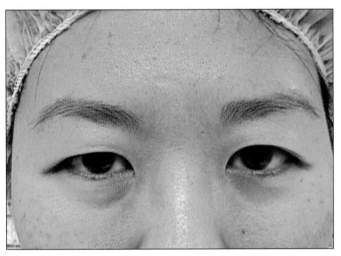

Figure 15.53

Commentary:

34 year old with hooding and single eyelid of the right and shielded with multiple creases over left side. The fissure size is smaller over the right side. Levator function: RUL 11mm, LUL 12mm. Intraoperatively: Tarsus measured 7mm. Used NTC shape and included 2.5mm skin. Myocutaneous flap excised; some fat excision. The crease formed well.

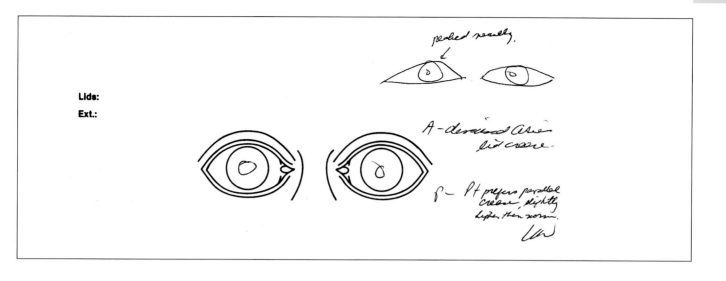

Lids:

Ext.:

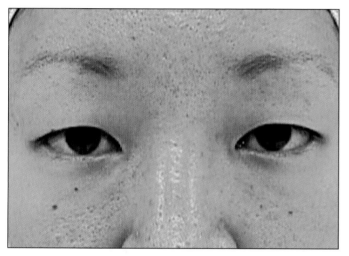

Figure 15.54

Commentary:

25 year old with single eyelid desires crease placement. Upper lid contour has slight peaking over medial one-third. Prefers higher-than-average parallel crease.

Intraoperatively: Tarsus measured 7mm. Designed a 7mm parallel crease shape. Had large amount of preaponeurotic fat, which was excised partially. A large roll of fatty infiltrate overlay the superior tarsal border and required clearance on each side for optimal crease formation.

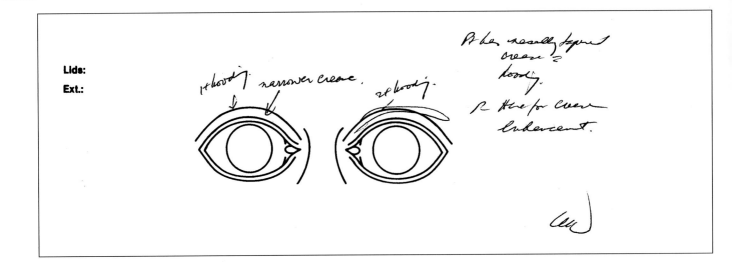

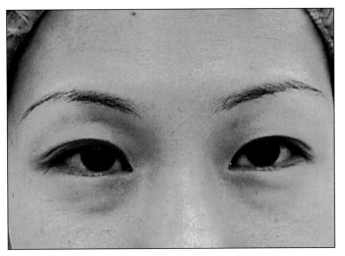

Figure 15.55

Commentary:

24 year old. Narrow crease with some shielding. RUL has shallower NTC; LUL has deeper-set low NTC. Desired crease enhancement. Intraoperatively: Tarsus measured 7.5mm. Used 7.5mm to design NTC with 2mm redundancy; excised fatty infiltrate along inferior edge of pretarsal orbicularis on both sides.

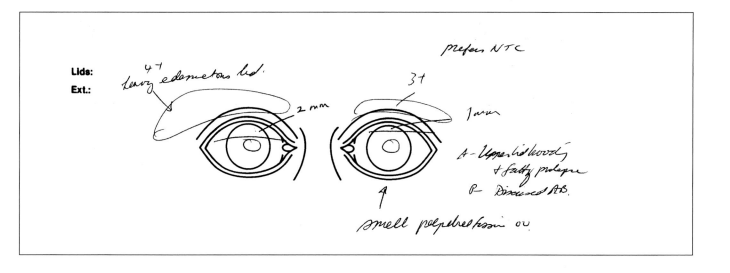

Lids:
Ext.:

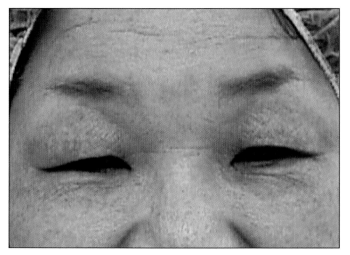

Figure 15.56

Commentary:

57-year-old patient with heavily hooded lid and fatty prolapse, more over the right side. RUL rest 2mm onto cornea. LUL rest 1mm. Has small palpebral fissure size bilaterally.

Intraoperatively: Could not evert tarsus to measure. Set crease at 7mm parallel shape. There was a large amount of amorphous fat inferior to the preaponeurotic fat, which in itself was inferiorly placed. Excised fat.

RUL – reinforce usual closure of 6-0 and 7-0 silk, with one double-armed 6-0 Vicryl passing from inferior pretarsal skin to aponeurosis.

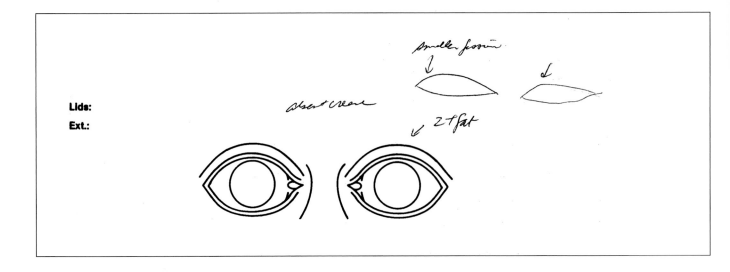

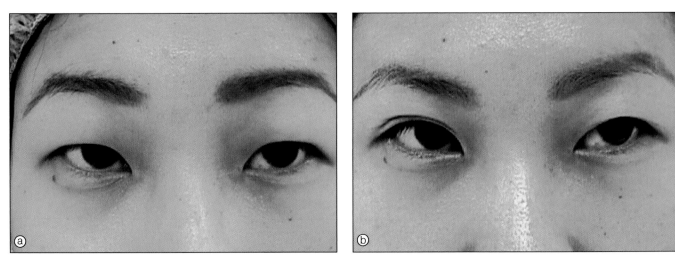

Figure 15.57 (a) Before and (b) one year after Asian blepharoplasty for crease enhancement over left upper lid.

Commentary:

23 year old with small palpebral fissure size, who is 1 year status post Asian blepharoplasty. Developed shallowing of crease over both upper eyelids.

RUL – tarsus measured 6.5 mm. Designed crease including less than 1mm of previous incision line. Lysed superior edge of incision through orbicularis. No unusual fat seen. Thick presence of preseptal orbicularis that was fluctuant was seen; this was excised.

LUL – crease was borderline after closure. Released the sutures and refixated by deeper placement onto aponeurosis. The medial portion of the levator aponeurosis appeared to have some fat infiltration.

REFERENCES

1. Chen WP. Asian blepharoplasty – anatomy and technique. J Ophthalmol Plast Reconstr Surg 1987;3:135–40.
2. Chen WP. A comparison of Caucasian and Asian blepharoplasty. Ophthalmic Pract 1991;9:216–22.
3. Chen WPD. Asian blepharoplasty: a surgical atlas. Newton, MA: Butterworth and Heinemann; 1995.
4. Chen WPD. Concept of triangular, rectangular and trapezoidal debulking of eyelid tissues: application in Asian blepharoplasty. Plast Reconstr Surg 1996;97:212–8.
5. Chen WPD. Eyelid and eyelid skin diseases. In: Lee D, Higginbotham E, eds. Clinical guide to comprehensive ophthalmology. New York: Thieme; 1998.
6. Chen WPD. Oculoplastic surgery: the essentials. New York: Thieme; 2001.
7. Chen WPD. Asian blepharoplasty: a surgical atlas. Newton: Butterworth–Heinemann; 1995.

Index